# ACL Reconstruction: Current Concepts

Steffen Sauer

# ACL Reconstruction: Current Concepts

Springer

Steffen Sauer
Aleris Hospital
Aarhus, Denmark

ISBN 978-3-031-68999-4 ISBN 978-3-031-69000-6 (eBook)
https://doi.org/10.1007/978-3-031-69000-6



This Springer imprint is published by the registered company Springer Nature Switzerland AG
The registered company address is: Gewerbestrasse 11, 6330 Cham, Switzerland

# Preface

More than 5000 years since the first known descriptions of the anterior cruciate ligament (ACL) from the Egyptian Smith papyrus, the ACL remains an enigmatic structure and is one of the most studied ligaments of the human body. The anatomical and biomechanical understanding of the ACL has constantly been refined based on a significant increase of scientific attention over the past decades. While only 133 studies were published on the ACL before 1979, almost 20,000 studies are available today. Surgical techniques have evolved in accordance with reliable hardware and sophisticated technology. However, the ongoing endeavour for ultimate improvement of ACL reconstruction outcomes seems to continue. The concept of ACL reconstruction seems to vacillate between a pragmatic anatomic approach and an evidence-based functional approach. The latter comprising the combination of ACL reconstruction and non-anatomical extra-articular functional procedures was once abandoned with emphasis on the importance of a well-performed anatomic ACL reconstruction without additional sources of morbidity. Currently, non-anatomical lateral extra-articular procedures are being reintroduced to improve the outcomes of ACL reconstruction. In future, the concept of ACL reconstruction will perhaps once again rest upon isolated anatomic ACL reconstruction once biological processes and mechanical alterations associated with ACL injury are well understood and newer ACL reconstruction techniques address individual morphology and insertional microarchitecture of the ACL. Modern technologies, high-quality research and systematic distribution of knowledge are thought to be fundamental for further improvement of ACL reconstruction outcomes in future. This comprehensive review invites the reader to delve into the fascinating world of ACL reconstructive surgery, elucidating important facts, but also drawing attention to unsolved questions and conflicting aspects.

Aarhus, Denmark
2024

Steffen Sauer

# Contents

# ACL Anatomy

## 1 Introduction

The anterior cruciate ligament (ACL) is currently described as an hour-glass shaped structure thought to be composed of an anteromedial (AMB) and posterolateral bundle (PLB) [8, 28]. The two bundles are thought to work reciprocally to restrain anterior tibial translation and internal tibial rotation [34]. In addition to resisting external forces, the ACL attunes physiological knee kinematics by centralising rotatory axes. In foetal stages, the anteromedial and posterolateral bundle are separated by a well-defined septum which embeds the supplying vasculature [10]. However, the foetal two-bundle entity of the ACL is not necessarily reflected in its adult microarchitecture. In the adult ACL, several non-parallel fibre-bundles compose a flat and rectangular core structure. In proximity to insertional areas, fibres diverge away from the core structure completing broad, bipartite insertion areas. On the femur, a thinner core structure insertion in line with the posterior cortex can be distinguished histologically from a broader fibrous fan-like insertion [47]. On the tibia, a c-shaped formation can be distinguished from a broader fan-like insertion, which completes the duck-foot appearance of the tibial insertion area [41]. The interface between core fibres and diverging fibres is characterised by a fold which deepens in knee flexion [27]. It has been hypothesised that the two-bundle appearance might represent an impression rather than an entity. Even though the ACL is thought to be a continuum of fibres with a gradient across the ligament, it is of biomechanical interest to distinguish an anteromedial from a posterolateral portion, as these portions inherit different biomechanical properties [45]. In synergy with the dynamic anatomic understanding of the knee, ACL reconstruction techniques have constantly been refined. There is a broad consensus among knee surgeons that deep understanding of the anatomy of the ACL is paramount for successful ACLR [32–34, 53]. However, the surgical term *anatomic ACL* does not refer to the anatomy of the ACL itself, as neither the unique macro-anatomy, the recruitment competent microanatomy, nor the multilayered transitional anchor architecture of the ACL are being addressed by modern

 
S. Sauer, *ACL Reconstruction: Current Concepts*,
https://doi.org/10.1007/978-3-031-69000-6_1

ACLR techniques. The term anatomic ACLR refers to graft positioning and volume. As arbitrary graft positioning within the broad native ACL insertion area does not necessarily ensure ACL graft longevity, the importance of reproducible anatomical descriptions of graft positioning in the scientific literature is currently emphasised. The ideal tunnel position within the ACL insertion area is still a matter of scientific debate. The anatomy of the ACL is still not fully charted and modern ACLR techniques fail to restore native biomechanics [53]. A trend is currently seen towards a more individual approach to ACLR, where the highly variable morphology of the ACL including its native length, course, dimension and insertional properties are taken into account.

## 2 Embryology

The ACL derives from blastemal cells in the embryological interzone and can be identified around the 7th week of gestation as a mesenchymal condensation [8]. By the 9th week of gestation, the ACL has the appearance of a cellular, oriented proliferation [55] and undergoes several modifications in the further course including enhanced fibre divergence, maturation and organised anchorage into the subchondral bone. The early and functional embryological formation of the ACL has led to the assumption that the morphological development of the knee is influenced by ACL-guided intrauterine knee kinematics. The embryologic ACL is surrounded by a mesentery-like synovial fold which carries the supplying vasculature. A well-defined septum between an anteromedial and a posterolateral bundle can be identified [10]. Agenesis of the posterolateral bundle has been observed, suggesting independent bundle development. In the course of embryogenic joint development, the ACL migrates into its more central position while preserving synovial coverage, thus remaining retro-synovial [8]. In addition, the lower extremities rotate 90 degrees internally into their final orientation, which has morphological and functional implications.

## 3 Anatomy

The ACL is currently described as an hour-glass shaped structure of dense connective tissue, thought to be composed of an anteromedial and posterolateral bundle [8, 12, 32–34]. Even though the foetal ACL has been shown to be separated by a well-defined septum [10], the two-bundle entity of the ACL is not necessarily reflected in its adult microarchitecture. The ACL is comprised of numerous twisted fascicles which form multiple multidirectional fibre bundles. The non-parallel fibre-bundles change their spatial inter-relationship, cross-sectional shape and size throughout their intra-articular course. Macroscopically, bundles can be identified and distinguished based on specific tension patterns. However, on a micro-structural level, the ACL is thought to represent a continuum of innumerous functional tissue-units, whose properties follow a linear gradient across the ligament [45]. It is of biomechanical interest to distinguish an anteromedial from a posterolateral portion, as these portions inherit different biomechanical properties [1, 14, 21, 44, 45]. The morphometrics of the ACL are highly variable [14] and in addition dependent on the flexion angle of the knee as length and width of the ACL behave reciprocally based on the effect of Poisson. The overall length of the ACL is thought to range between 22 and 41 mm [7]. The isolated average length of the AMB and PLB have been described to measure 33 and 18 mm, respectively [43]. The overall width of the ACL has been described to range from 7 to 12 mm. The cross-sectional area and volume of the ACL have been described to range between 30 to 53 $mm^2$, and 854 to 1858 $mm^3$ respectively [7]. Males show a larger absolute ACL volume compared to females with 1712.2 and 1200.1 $mm^3$, respectively. The thinnest part of the ACL is typically found at an average of approximately 46 percent of the distance from the femoral insertion centre to the tibial insertion centre. It has been found to measure 33 and 38 $mm^2$ for females and males, respectively. The cross-sectional area of the ACL mid-portion increases towards the insertion sites. Close to the femoral insertion, the cross section has been found to be 52 and 55 $mm^2$ for females and males, respectively. Based on the effect of Poisson, the length and cross-sectional area behave reciprocally, thus the cross-sectional area of the ACL decreases with increasing length during knee extension. The shortest length and consecutive largest diameter of the ACL isthmus are found in 90 degrees of flexion. The macro-anatomy of the ACL has been thoroughly revisited but tends to be subjected to morphological variability as several factors influence the macroscopic appearance of the ACL. Regarding cadaveric descriptions, the age of the specimen and associated degenerative processes, the dissecting technique as well as the knee flexion angle in which the specimen is prepared, have been shown to influence the appearance of the ACL. The in-vivo appearance of the ACL is influenced by the degree of knee flexion, as well as by its twisted surface membrane and variable arrangement of connective tissue. In extension, the ACL appears straight. In flexion, as the distal femoral portion of the ACL insertion is brought forward, a noticeable fold is created, hereby eventually enhancing the impression of distinguishable bundles [27]. If the surface membrane is removed, the ACL has a rather flat, rectangular ribbon-like appearance, and has been described as to resemble *lasagna* [26, 42]. The relatively thin ribbon-like mid-portion of the ACL stands in contrast to its broader, bipartite insertion areas, which complete the hour-glass shape of the ACL [46–48]. The mean length and width of the ribbon-like mid-portion has been described to measure 11.4 and 3.4 mm, respectively. However, the cross-section of the ACL corpus is not a simple geometrical form and changes dimension depending on the cross-sectional level. The cross-section of the ACL entails fibres which form direct insertion areas as well as fibres which form fan-like insertional extensions [47]. On the medial aspect of the lateral femoral condyle, portions of the mid-substance fibres of the ACL insert along the intercondylar femoral ridge (Resident's ridge) in a long but relatively thin formation. Identical fibres diverge posteriorly towards the femoral cartilage and form a broad fibrous extension, which completes the ovoid femoral insertion site. The area of the femoral ACL insertion is highly variable [20, 35, 49] and has been described to range between 60 and 130 $mm^2$ [36]. Its biconvex boundaries are the slightly curved femoral intercondylar ridge [5] (which is in line with the posterior femoral cortex) and the posterior articular margin of the lateral condyle [6, 19]. The femoral insertion site comprises direct and indirect insertions covering AMB and PLB positions [40]. The insertion of the AMB and PLB are inconsistently separated by the bifurcate ridge. The mean areas of the direct and indirect insertion of the AM bundle have been described to range between 26–63 mm$^2$ and 10–35 mm$^2$, respectively, depending on age and gender. The mean areas of the direct and indirect insertion of the PL bundle have been described to range between 24–51 mm$^2$ and 10–34 mm$^2$, respectively, depending on age and gender [29]. The direct insertion along the femoral intercondylar ridge is composed of fibres which enter the bone almost perpendicularly through a complex multilayered anchor-architecture involving mineralised and non-mineralised cartilaginous layers [16]. In contrast, the fibrous extensional fibres are attached more loosely and parallel to the bone, lacking a transitional zone. Fibres of the mid-substance change orientation in knee motion, while fan-like extensional fibres remain unchanged in respect to their femoral surface orientation. In knee flexion, the mid-substance fibres are bent and folded over fan-like extensional fibres. Fibrocartilaginous zones of the direct insertion are believed to control this mechanism. The proportional contribution of direct fibres to the entire femoral insertion site ranges from under 20 percent to over 50 percent. Accordingly, the width of the direct insertion site is subjected to variability and has been reported by Iwahashi and Sasaki to measure 5.3 and 8.0 mm, respectively [16, 37]. The indirect insertion site has a membrane-like appearance and is formed by fibres which diverge posteriorly towards the posterior femoral cartilage. The 2-phase anchor-architecture comprises superficial fibres which are connected to the periosteum as well as deep fibres which are connected to the bone [17]. The interdigitation of the anchor-architecture is less deep compared to direct insertion. A cartilaginous zone is lacking. Posteriorly, fibres blend into the posterior femoral cartilage, as seen on immunohistological observations. While direct fibres are thought to be the primary restraint to tensile forces, indirect fibres are thought to be involved in controlling shear forces. The interface between direct and indirect fibres is characterised by a fold, which deepens in higher flexion angles [27]. Insertional areas are thought to comprise a continuum of bundle-formations which become progressively loaded depending on knee flexion and femoro-tibial alignment. The appearance of the tibial ACL insertion is associated with significant variability but typically described as an oval, triangular or c-shaped formation, bounded posteriorly by the medial and lateral intercondylar tubercles, anteriorly by the Parson's knob, medially by the medial intercondylar ridge and laterally by the anterior horn of the lateral meniscus [54]. The Parson's knob (tuberculum intercondylare tertium [4]) is thought to represent a bony ridge-like elevation [31]. The tibial insertion site is thought to comprise two bundle areas. The crescent shaped anteromedial insertion area is located along an L-shaped formation constituted by the Parson's knob and the medial intercondylar ridge, enfolding the smaller PL insertion area which is located diametrically close to the lateral tibial spine. The resulting division between bundles has a posteromedial-to-anterolateral curved course [18]. The centre of the tibial insertion site is thought to be located 10.5 mm posterior to the Parson's knob,

13 mm anterior to the retro-eminence ridge and 7.5 mm medial to the anterior horn of the lateral meniscus [22]. The anterior aspect of the anterior horn of the lateral meniscus is thought to be in line with the AM bundle [39]. The fibrous attachments of the posterior aspect of the anterior horn of the lateral meniscus are thought to be in line with the PL bundle. The anterior inter-meniscal ligament is located 9.1 mm anterior from the centre of the tibial insertion area. The ACL insertion is located 7 mm anterior to the PCL. Several anatomical studies with emphasis on meticulous removal of synovial coverage and connective tissue have failed to identify a functional posterolateral portion of the ACL and describe the tibial insertion area as a continuous c-shaped, Cc-shaped or j-shaped anteromedial insertion [42, 47]. Direct fibres form a curved narrow anteromedial insertion along the medial intercondylar ridge and the Parson's Knob while indirect fibres extend anteriorly to complete the 3-dimensional duck-foot appearance of the tibial ACL insertion site. The bony floor of the tibial insertion area is a 3-dimensional *relief* rather than a flat surface. As seen on sagittal images, the insertion area lies immersed posterior to the Parson's knob. The recently discovered central intercondylar ridge bisects the slope of the medial intercondylar ridge between the tibial insertion of the anterior cruciate ligament and anterior horn of lateral meniscus [22, 54]. Both the anterior and posterior horn of the lateral meniscus blend into the crescent formation of the tibial ACL insertion area, which has implications for ACL resistance behaviour based on meniscal movement and position. Observing tibial plateaus from TKA surgery (Fig. 1), the ACL insertion area and the surrounding connective tissue show substantial diversity. Even though only limited conclusions can be drawn based on the degenerative nature of the tibial plateaus, the potential benefit of individualised ACL reconstruction techniques may become evident.

The function of the ACL is typically explained through a simplified two-bundle model, where an anteromedial and posterolateral bundle are distinguished [23]. Bundle nomenclature is based on tibial insertional morphology [1]. Direct and indirect insertions are not considered. Even though newest research indicates synergistic bundle behaviour, it is currently believed that the AM and PL bundle work reciprocally. The AM bundle is hereby believed to act as the primary restraint against anterior tibial translation in higher flexion angles, while the PL bundle acts as the primary restraint against anterior tibial translation and rotational torque towards full knee extension. Accordingly, the AM and PL bundle are thought to reach their maximal lengths in flexion and extension, respectively. However, there is conflicting evidence regarding exact length-patterns of the AMB and PLB. When termination points are being specified within insertional areas, the AMB and PLB elongate in parallel as the knee is extended [9], indicating synergy. The femoral condyles comprise more than one rotational axis. In addition, femoro-tibial alignment is dynamically altered during knee movement. Accordingly, the force vector changes with every degree of knee flexion. Altering fibre configurations within the ACL ensure multi-planar stability. To date, there is also inconclusive evidence regarding the exact contribution of the AM and PL bundle in terms of stability. Several cadaveric studies have failed to show a significant difference in knee kinematics with isolated AM or PL bundle deficiency, concluding that significant knee laxity must comprise injury to both bundles. In more recent approaches, the ACL has been reviewed based on functional areas and corresponding histological architecture. The broad cylindrical insertion sites are exposed to overlapping shear, tensile and compression forces and display an underlying complex multilayered microarchitecture including a fibrocartilaginous layer which is thought to control fibre bending. The thin mid-portion of the ACL resists mainly tensile forces which is reflected in high fibre density with recruitment competent arrangement. An anterior fibrocartilage portion, similar to tendons passing a pulley, resists compression forces induced by the femoral notch. The anatomy of the ACL is not fully charted, and the anatomic understanding of the ACL as well as deriving surgical techniques will certainly be refined in the future. Whether the implantation of an ACL-allograft with retained anchor-architecture is beneficial remains currently unclear.

## 4 Histology

The ACL is composed of fibroblasts which provide the extracellular matrix (ECM) by secreting fibrous proteins and ground substance. Fibroblasts are capable of locomotion by means of an actin-based cytoskeleton [25]. Ground substance is composed of water, glycosaminoglycans (GAG), proteoglycans and adhesion proteins and has several functions such as the storage of water, the exchange of materials as well as the binding of components of the ground substance to one another and to the surface of the cells. In addition, ground substance controls the metabolic activity as well as the shape of the tissue [25]. The most common fibrous protein is pro-collagen which is secreted into the ECM and aggregated into larger cross-linked collagen formations. From the nearly 30 collagen-types currently known, collagen I, II, III, IV, IX and X are thought to play important roles in the ACL. The common structural nature of all collagen types is the presence of a triple coiled-coil right-handed helix, constituted by three polypeptide chains with a glycine residue in every third position [24]. The diversity is based mainly on these helically arranged protein chains (alpha chains), isoforms and supramolecular structures. Type I collagen, which is the most abundant fibre in the ACL, is composed of three diverse alpha chains, while collagen type III is composed of 3 identical alpha chains. The cartilage-typical type II collagen is composed of two identical and one diverse alpha chain. Type II and III collagen are found at the ACL insertion sites, indicating the presence of shear forces and intrinsic healing potential. Collagen type I forms the fibril, which is the base-unit of the hierarchical architecture of the ACL. Fibrils can be differentiated into two types of fibrils dependent on their morphology and purpose. Fibrils with a smooth outline ensure the three-dimensional organisation of the ligament [51]. Fibrils which are produced by fibroblasts, have an irregular outline and resist loading. The specific elongation and resistance pattern of fibrils is dependent on their crimp geometry. Straight or planar sinusoidal fibrils are mainly found in the centre of the ACL and rapidly resist loading. Fibrils organised in a cylindrical helical manner are typically found in the periphery of the ACL and are first gradually straightened out by increasing forces before resisting loading. These fibres are "recruited" gradually under increasing tensile forces to increase the tissue resistance and tensile strength. Fibrils form fibre bundles which are surrounded by the endoligament to form a subfascicular unit. Several subfasciculi are contained by the periligament and form twisted fascicles [38]. Numerous fascicles and the supplying vasculature are surrounded by the epiligament and covered by the subintima and intima of the synovial layer. The femoral and tibial ACL insertion areas display a multilayered, asymmetric and polar microarchitecture intended to resist multiaxial loading. Different parts of the insertion area show characteristic properties based on the underlying histological composition. The complexity of the insertion areas with a specific tissue gradient does not only increase the susceptibility to injury but represents a major challenge regarding ACL reconstruction. Particularly, portions of the PL bundle are susceptible to injury in landing manoeuvres. The ACL can microscopically be differentiated into 3 main parts, primarily based on composition and resulting consistency: the proximal part, the ACL corpus and the distal part. The proximal part comprises the femoral insertion site which can be differentiated into direct and indirect insertion areas. The direct fibre insertion is characterised by fibres which enter the bone almost perpendicularly through a 4-layer anchor architecture with a linear tissue resistance gradient [11]. The first layer is the ligamentous layer which is composed of elongated, partly ovoid ligamentocytes and collagen type I. The second layer is the non-calcified fibrocartilage layer which is composed of ovoid fibro-chondrocytes and collagen type I, II and IX. The third layer is the calcified fibrocartilage layer composed of round fibro-chondrocytes and collagen type I, II and X as well as hydroxyapatite. The fourth layer is the bone transition layer composed of osteoblast, osteoclasts, osteocytes, collagen I and hydroxyapatite. The interfaces between the zones are characterised by interdigitations, which increase the contact interface and consecutive resistance. Between layer II and III, an acellular tidemark formation can be identified. The tidemark formation is composed mainly of phospholipids and represents a nutritious supply barrier. While layer II is supplied by the vasculature of the ACL, layer III is supplied by the vasculature of the bone. In contrast to direct fibres, indirect fibres are attached to the bone in a more parallel manner through a simpler 2-layer anchor architecture. Superficial fibres are hereby attached to the periosteum and deep fibres are attached directly to the bone. A transitional zone is lacking and the interdigitation is less aggressive compared to the direct insertion site. While tensile resistance is mainly ascribed direct fibres, indirect fibres are hypothesised to be involved in attuning ligament mechanisms and control shear forces. The continuum of direct fibres, covering the AM bundle and PL bundle areas, display a linear tissue gradient with increased percentage of calcified and non-calcified fibrocartilage towards the AMB. In addition, the AMB area shows stronger interdigitations and more uniform fibre alignment compared to the PL bundle area, indicating significant force exposure. This is also underlined by the highly attuned spatial orientation of the femoral trabeculae and the fibres of the ACL at the proximal posterior part of the femoral insertion. The mid-portion of the ACL shows high density of collagen and low cellularity. Fibres show specific crimp geometry and are recruited by progressive loading, hereby increasing tissue stiffness and tensile resistance. The anterior portion of the ACL is characterised by collagen fibres and fibroblasts which form a cartilage and fibrocartilage section. These cartilage and fibrocartilage sections are typically found in tendons passing a pulley [15]. The distal part of the ACL comprises the tibial insertion site. Even though the tibial insertion site resembles the femoral insertion site, there are significant differences. The calcified and non-calcified layers of the 4-layered architecture are significantly thinner compared to the corresponding femoral layers and fibres are generally attached in a more obtuse angle compared to the femoral attachment. The parallelism of the tibial trabeculae and the fibres of the ACL is exceptional, indicating exposure to predominantly unidirectional force.

## 5 ACL Innervation

The innervation of the ACL is provided through posterior articular branches of the tibial nerve which penetrate the posterior aspect of the joint capsule [29]. The majority of nerve fibres accompany vessels to control vasomotor function. The remaining nerve fibres are involved in proprioception through mechanoreceptors as well as nociception through unmyelinated free nerve endings. Mechanoreceptors have different functions and are accordingly positioned with high density typically near the femoral and tibial insertion sites [3]. Ruffini receptors perceive elongation and are located predominantly at the upper/femoral part of the ACL where substantial ligamentous deformity takes place. Vater–Pacini receptors perceive speed and acceleration and are located at the femoral and tibial ends of the ACL. Golgi-like receptors perceive tension and are located near the ACL attachment site as well as superficially beneath the synovial membrane of the ACL. Free-nerve endings ensure nociception. The mechanoreceptors represent the afferent arc of the ACL reflex. Following the activation of these receptors, the efferent arc of the reflex cycle is carried by the output of muscle spindles through the fusimotor system. The ACL reflex is not regarded as a protective mechanism as more than 100 ms typically elapse before relevant stabilising muscle force can be established while the ground reaction force may induce femoro-tibial subluxation and ACL rupture in under 40 ms. However, the ACL reflex is an essential part of normal knee kinematics and muscle programs. For instance, the maximal voluntary contraction exertion of the quadriceps femoris is dependent on the function of the mechanoreceptors. Loss of extension following ACLR is typically based on lack of afferent feedback or over-activation of mechanical receptors of the PCL impeding normal muscle function. ACL Remnant preservation under ACLR may increase the chance of a functioning ACL reflex and has been associated with superior clinical outcomes [52].

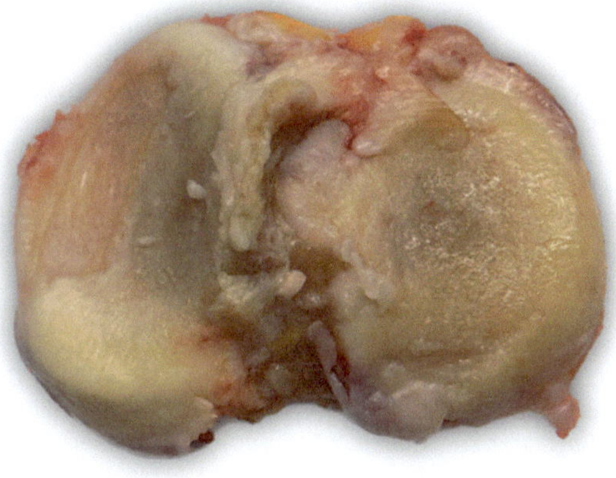

**Fig. 1** Tibial plateau from TKA surgery

## 6 ACL Vasculature

The blood supply of the ACL is established through the middle genicular artery (MGA), which is a branch from the popliteal artery. Following joint access through the posterior capsule, the MGA divides into an epiphyseal branch and a ligamentous branch. The ligamentous branch arborizes into a superficial network-like system located beneath the synovial part which anastomoses with terminal branches of the medial inferior genicular artery to complete the network-like vasculature [50]. These periligamentous vessels penetrate the ACL perpendicularly and communicate with an endoligamentous network which represents the inner pendant to the outer network [2, 8]. The inner vasculature does not communicate beyond the ACL insertion sites which has implications for ligamentous healing potential. The density of the vasculature is higher in the proximal/femoral part of the ACL compared to the distal/tibial part. In addition, the proximal portion of the ACL is supported by collateral branches of arteries directed to the roof of the intercondylar notch and the lateral femoral condyle. A minor amount of blood is supplied to the distal portion of the ACL through infrapatellar branches of the inferior genicular artery. The periligamentous fold of vessels is absent in a small zone approximately 5–10 mm proximal to the tibial attachment. The anterior fibrocartilaginous part of the tissue is avascular, indicating the presence of compressive forces. Some properties of the ACL ensure homeostasis rather than biomechanical performance.

## References


1. Amis A, Dawkins G. Functional anatomy of the anterior cruciate ligament. Fibre bundle actions related to ligament replacements and injuries. J Bone Joint Surg. 1991;73 (British volume).
2. Arnoczky SP. Anatomy of the anterior cruciate ligament. Clin Orthop Relat Res. 1983;172.

3. Banios K, Raoulis V, Fyllos A, Chytas D, Mitrousias V, Zibis A. Anterior and Posterior Cruciate Ligaments Mechanoreceptors: A Review of Basic Science. Diagnostics (Basel) 2022;12. https://doi.org/10.3390/diagnostics12020331
4. Berg EE. Parsons' Knob (Tuberculum Intercondylare Tedium): A Guide to Tibial Anterior Cruciate Ligament Insertion. Clin Orthopaed Relat Res. 1993;292.
5. Bicer EK, Lustig S, Servien E, Selmi TA, Neyret P. Current knowledge in the anatomy of the human anterior cruciate ligament. Knee Surg Sports Traumatol Arthrosc. 2010;18.
6. Colombet P, Robinson J, Christel P, Franceschi JP, Djian P, Bellier G, et al. Morphology of anterior cruciate ligament attachments for anatomic reconstruction: a cadaveric dissection and radiographic study. Arthroscopy. 2006;22.
7. Cone SG, Howe D, Fisher MB. Size and shape of the human anterior cruciate ligament and the impact of sex and skeletal growth: a systematic review. JBJS Rev. 2019;7(6): e8.
8. Duthon VB, Barea C, Abrassart S, Fasel JH, Fritschy D, Menetrey J. Anatomy of the anterior cruciate ligament. Knee Surg Sports Traumatol Arthrosc. 2006;14.
9. Englander ZA, Garrett WE, Spritzer CE, DeFrate LE. In vivo attachment site to attachment site length and strain of the ACL and its bundles during the full gait cycle measured by MRI and high-speed biplanar radiography. J Biomech 2020;98:109443. https://doi.org/10.1016/j.jbiomech.2019.109443
10. Ferretti M, Ekdahl M, Shen W, Fu FH. Osseous landmarks of the femoral attachment of the anterior cruciate ligament: an anatomic study. Arthroscopy. 2007;23.
11. Fu FH, Bennett, Craig H, Lattermann, Christian, Ma C. Benjamin. Current Trends in Anterior Cruciate Ligament Reconstruction. The American Journal of Sports Medicine 1999;27:821–30. https://doi.org/10.1177/03635465990270062501
12. Fu FH, Shen W, Starman JS, Okeke N, Irrgang JJ. Primary anatomic double-bundle anterior cruciate ligament reconstruction: a preliminary 2-year prospective study. Am J Sports Med. 2008;36.
13. George Chahla and Robert Laprade 2017. 2-Anatomy-of-the-ACL-Insertions.
14. Girgis FG, Marshall JL, Monajem AL. The cruciate ligaments of the knee joint. Anatomical, functional and experimental analysis. Clin Orthop Relat Res. 1975;106.
15. Gögele C, Hahn J, Schulze-Tanzil G. Anatomical Tissue Engineering of the Anterior Cruciate Ligament Entheses. Int J Mol Sci 2023;24. https://doi.org/10.3390/ijms241119745
16. Iwahashi T, Shino K, Nakata K, Otsubo H, Suzuki T, Amano H, et al. Direct anterior cruciate ligament insertion to the femur assessed by histology and 3-dimensional volume-rendered computed tomography. Arthroscopy. 2010;26.
17. Jorge PB, Escudeiro D, Severino NR, Santili C, de Paula Leite Cury R, Junior AD, Guglielmetti LGB. Positioning of the femoral tunnel in anterior cruciate ligament reconstruction: functional anatomical reconstruction. BMJ Open Sport Exerc Med 2018;4:e000420. https://doi.org/10.1136/bmjsem-2018-000420
18. Jorge C, Robert F. LaPrade: Anatomy of the ACL Insertions: Arthroscopic Identification of the Attachments © ISAKOS 2017 173 N. Nakamura et al. (eds.), Controversies in the Technical Aspects of ACL Reconstruction. https://doi.org/10.1007/978-3-662-52742-9_17
19. Kim YM, Joo YB, Lee KY, Hwang SJ. Femoral footprint for anatomical single-bundle anterior cruciate ligament reconstruction: a cadaveric study. Knee Surg Relat Res. 2018;30.
20. Kopf S, Pombo MW, Szczodry M, Irrgang JJ, Fu FH. Size variability of the human anterior cruciate ligament insertion sites. Am J Sports Med. 2011;39.
21. Kraeutler MJ, Wolsky RM, Vidal AF, Bravman JT. Anatomy and biomechanics of the native and reconstructed anterior cruciate ligament: surgical implications. J Bone Joint Surg Am. 2017;99.
22. LaPrade CM, Ellman MB, Rasmussen MT, James EW, Wijdicks CA, Engebretsen L. Anatomy of the anterior root attachments of the medial and lateral menisci: a quantitative analysis. Am J Sports Med. 2014;42.
23. Luites JWH, Wymenga AB, Blankevoort L, Kooloos JGM. Description of the attachment geometry of the anteromedial and posterolateral bundles of the ACL from arthroscopic perspective for anatomical tunnel placement. Knee Surg Sports Traumatol Arthrosc. 2007;15(12):1422–31.

24. Makareeva, Elena, Leikin, Sergey. Chapter 7 - Collagen Structure, Folding and Function. Osteogenesis Imperfecta. San Diego: Academic Press, 2014;pp. 71–84. https://www.sciencedirect.com/science/article/pii/B9780123971654000071
25. Marieswaran M, Jain I, Garg B, Sharma V, Kalyanasundaram D. A Review on Biomechanics of Anterior Cruciate Ligament and Materials for Reconstruction. Appl Bionics Biomech 2018;4657824. https://doi.org/10.1155/2018/4657824
26. Mochizuki T, Fujishiro H, Nimura A, Mahakkanukrauh P, Yasuda K, Muneta T, et al. Anatomic and histologic analysis of the mid-substance and fan-like extension fibres of the anterior cruciate ligament during knee motion, with special reference to the femoral attachment. Knee Surg Sport Traumatol Arthrosc Off J ESSKA. 2013;22.
27. Mochizuki T, Fujishiro H, Nimura A, Mahakkanukrauh P, Yasuda K, Muneta T, et al. Anatomic and histologic analysis of the mid-substance and fan-like extension fibres of the anterior cruciate ligament during knee motion, with special reference to the femoral attachment. Knee Surg Sports Traumatol Arthrosc. 2014;22.
28. Mochizuki T, Muneta T, Nagase T, Shirasawa S, Akita KI, Sekiya I. Cadaveric knee observation study for describing anatomic femoral tunnel placement for two-bundle anterior cruciate ligament reconstruction. Arthroscopy. 2006;22.
29. Morales-Avalos R, Castillo-Escobedo TA, Elizondo-Omaña RE, Del Carmen Theriot-Giron M, Perelli S, Guzmán-López S, Peña-Martínez VM, Vílchez-Cavazos F, Monllau JC. The morphology of the tibial footprint of the anterior cruciate ligament changes with ageing from oval/elliptical to C-shaped. Knee Surg Sports Traumatol Arthrosc 2021;29:922–30. https://doi.org/10.1007/s00167-020-06049-7
30. Morales-Avalos R, Torres-González EM, Padilla-Medina JR, Monllau JC. ACL anatomy: Is there still something to learn?. Revista Española de Cirugía Ortopédica y Traumatología. 2023. https://doi.org/10.1016/j.recot.2023.02.005. https://www.sciencedirect.com/science/article/pii/S188844152300070X
31. Nishimori M, Furuta T, Deie M. Parsons' knob, the bony landmark of the tibial insertion of the anterior cruciate ligament, evaluated by three-dimensional computed tomography. Asia-Pacific J Sports Med Arthrosc Rehabil Technol. 2014;1(4):126–31.
32. Norwood LA, Cross MJ. Anterior cruciate ligament: functional anatomy of its bundles in rotatory instabilities. Am J Sports Med. 1979;7.
33. Odensten M, Gillquist J. Functional anatomy of the anterior cruciate ligament and a rationale for reconstruction. J Bone Joint Surg Am. 1985;67.
34. Petersen W, Zantop T. Anatomy of the anterior cruciate ligament with regard to its two bundles. Clin Orthop Relat Res. 2007;454.
35. Piefer JW, Pflugner TR, Hwang MD, Lubowitz JH. Anterior cruciate ligament femoral footprint anatomy: systematic review of the 21st century literature. Arthroscopy. 2012;28.
36. Runer A, Keeling L, Wagala N, Nugraha H, Özbek EA, Hughes JD, et al. Current trends in graft choice for anterior cruciate ligament reconstruction—part I: anatomy, biomechanics, graft incorporation and fixation. J Exp Orthop. 2023;10(1):37.
37. Sasaki N, Ishibashi Y, Tsuda E, Yamamoto Y, Maeda S, Mizukami H, et al. The femoral insertion of the anterior cruciate ligament: discrepancy between macroscopic and histological observations. Arthroscopy. 2012;28(8):1135–46.
38. Schulze-Tanzil G. Intraarticular Ligament Degeneration Is Interrelated with Cartilage and Bone Destruction in Osteoarthritis. Cells. 2019;8. https://doi.org/10.3390/cells8090990
39. Siebold R, Ellert T, Metz S, Metz J. Tibial insertions of the anteromedial and posterolateral bundles of the anterior cruciate ligament: morphometry, arthroscopic landmarks, and orientation model for bone tunnel placement. Arthroscopy. 2008;24.
40. Siebold R, Ellert T, Metz S, Metz J. Femoral insertions of the anteromedial and posterolateral bundles of the anterior cruciate ligament: morphometry and arthroscopic orientation models for double-bundle bone tunnel placement—a cadaver study. Arthroscopy. 2008;24.
41. Siebold R, Schuhmacher P, Fernandez F, Śmigielski R, Fink C, Brehmer A, et al. Flat midsubstance of the anterior cruciate ligament with tibial "C"-shaped insertion site. Knee Surg Sports Traumatol Arthrosc. 2015;23(11):3136–42.

42. Siebold R, Schuhmacher P, Fernandez F, Śmigielski R, Fink C, Brehmer A, Kirsch J. Flat midsubstance of the anterior cruciate ligament with tibial "C"-shaped insertion site. Knee Surg Sports Traumatol Arthrosc. 2014. https://doi.org/10.1007/s00167-014-3058-6.
43. Siegel L, Vandenakker-Albanese C, Siegel D. Anterior cruciate ligament injuries: anatomy, physiology, biomechanics, and management. Clin J Sport Med Off J Can Acad Sport Med. 2012;22:349–55.
44. Skelley NW, Castile RM, Cannon PC, Weber CI, Brophy RH, Lake SP. Regional variation in the mechanical and microstructural properties of the human anterior cruciate ligament. Am J Sports Med. 2016;44.
45. Skelley NW, Lake SP, Brophy RH. Microstructural properties of the anterior cruciate ligament. Ann Joint. 2017;2.
46. Śmigielski R, Zdanowicz U, Drwiega M, Ciszek B, Ciszkowska-Lyson B, Siebold R. Ribbon like appearance of the midsubstance fibres of the anterior cruciate ligament close to its femoral insertion site: a cadaveric study including 111 knees. Knee Surg Sports Traumatol Arthrosc. 2015;23.
47. Śmigielski R, Zdanowicz U, Drwiega M, Ciszek B, Ciszkowska-Lyson B, Siebold R. Ribbon like appearance of the midsubstance fibres of the anterior cruciate ligament close to its femoral insertion site: a cadaveric study including 111 knees. Knee Surg Sports Traumatol Arthrosc. 2014. https://doi.org/10.1007/s00167-014-3146-7.
48. Śmigielski R, Zdanowicz U, Drwiega M, Ciszek B, Williams A. The anatomy of the anterior cruciate ligament and its relevance to the technique of reconstruction. Bone Joint J. 2016;98-B.
49. Takahashi M, Doi M, Abe M, Suzuki D, Nagano A. Anatomical study of the femoral and tibial insertions of the anteromedial and posterolateral bundles of human anterior cruciate ligament. Am J Sports Med. 2006;34.
50. Toy BJ, Yeasting RA, Morse DE, McCann P. Arterial supply to the human anterior cruciate ligament. J Athl Train. 1995;30:149–52.
51. Wan C, Hao Z, Wen S. A review on research on development of ligament constitutive relations on macro, meso, and micro levels. Acta Mech Solida Sin. 2013;26:331–43.
52. Wang HD, Wang FS, Gao SJ, Zhang YZ. Remnant preservation technique versus standard technique for anterior cruciate ligament reconstruction: a meta-analysis of randomized controlled trials. J Orthop Surg Res 2018;13:231. https://doi.org/10.1186/s13018-018-0937-4.
53. Woo SL, Wu C, Dede O, Vercillo F, Noorani S. Biomechanics and anterior cruciate ligament reconstruction. J Orthop Surg Res. 2006;1:2.
54. Yonetani Y, Kusano M, Tsujii A, Kinugasa K, Hamada M, Shino K. Tibial insertion of the anterior cruciate ligament and anterior horn of the lateral meniscus share the lateral slope of the medial intercondylar ridge: A computed tomography study in a young, healthy population. Knee. 2019;26(3):612–8.
55. Yoo H, Marappa-Ganeshan R. Anatomy, Bony Pelvis and Lower Limb, Knee Anterior Cruciate Ligament. StatPearls. Treasure Island (FL): StatPearls Publishing

# ACL Biomechanics

## 1 Introduction

Biomechanics, i.e., the observation of biological systems from a mechanical perspective, is typically described through kinetics and kinematics. While the term kinetics refers to the relationship between motion and its causes, specifically forces and torque, kinematics describes the 3-dimensional geometry of a motion regarding displacement, acceleration and velocity. The composition of a ligament defines its kinetic properties, e.g. maximal load to failure and young's modulus. The kinetic properties and orientation of a ligament have implications for joint kinematics. Biomechanical problem formulations have been addressed by several approaches including in vivo kinematic data, robotic testing and computational modelling analyses [3, 10, 13, 14, 17, 26, 47, 55, 74, 88]. The inherent biomechanics of the knee joint are complex and not yet fully elucidated. As a result, there is conflicting evidence in the literature concerning the biomechanical function and nature of the ACL. Historically, the function of the ACL is simplified to the restrain of anterior tibial translation and internal tibial rotation. However, the ACL is also thought to be involved in the stabilisation and centralization of rotational axes and the balance of stability while allowing a variable degree of physiological rotatory laxity. Indisputable, however, is the fact that the ACL is of paramount importance for knee biomechanics [9, 11], which is reflected in the fact that ACL transection is used to reliably induce osteoarthritis in experimental animal studies. It is assumed that ACL deficiency is associated with altered biomechanics, placing excessive stress on supporting structures. The clinical scope of the biomechanical alteration is to some extent dependent on the individual's response and remains unpredictable.

 
S. Sauer, *ACL Reconstruction: Current Concepts*,
https://doi.org/10.1007/978-3-031-69000-6_2

## 2 Kinetics

The kinetic behaviour of a ligament is based on several factors including the corresponding histology and microarchitecture. The ACL comprises several areas which are composed specifically to withstand different types of forces. The anterior cartilaginous portion of the ACL, which encounters the intercondylar notch, withstands compression forces (perpendicular forces). The ACL insertional areas with a direct 4-layered and indirect 2-layered anchor architecture withstand overlapping tensile (longitudinal) and shear forces (parallel forces). The ACL corpus with high fibre density and unique recruitment competent crimp geometry withstands tensile forces (longitudinal forces). Forces and their deformational impact can be described by stress and strain. Stress is hereby defined as the amount of loading per square millimetre of cross-sectional area. The resulting deformation is defined as strain and expressed unit-less as the percentage of deformation [115]. As unidirectional stress induces 3-dimensional deformation, ligaments have a characteristic Poisson's ratio [100, 111] which describes the ratio of lateral and axial deformation. This may explain why ACL length and diameter behave reciprocally. Ligaments show a specific stress–strain association. The stress–strain curve of the ACL can be divided into four areas [87]. The toe-area of the curve is the result of forces which straighten out fibril crimp without significant ligamentous strain. Once fibril crimp is increasingly straightened out and numerous fibrils are recruited, fibrils undergo reversible elastic deformation which is reflected in the second, quasilinear area of the curve. When the maximal reversible elongation of the ACL is reached, the slope of the curve decreases while plastic fibril deformation takes place. The last, suddenly decreasing area of the curve represents the complete failure of the bone-ligament-bone complex. Based on the slope of the linear portion of the curve, ACL stiffness can be derived, which corresponds to the forces acting on the ACL. The ACL is thought to restrain anterior tibial translation, which is based on the observation that transection of the ACL induces increased anteroposterior laxity. However, pure anterior tibial translation does rarely occur physiologically. The femoro-tibial displacement is the result of poly-centric rotation, and the ACL is thought to be involved in the control of rotational movements and maintenance of rotational axes. As a result, the contribution of the ACL to resisting forced anterior tibial translation decreases significantly when the knee is unconstrained. The ACL is thought to display a dynamic functional isometry. Even though no true isometry is found in the ACL, altering recruitment competent fibre-constellations can maintain a constant or progressively changing resistance through knee motion. Forces on the ACL are potentiated by knee abduction and internal/external rotation. The force which is developed within a ligament as a response to external force, is defined as the in-situ force. The in-situ force (N), being a vector, has a point of application, magnitude and direction and can exceed the applied external force [47]. The in-situ force can be determined by different means, e.g., a strain gauge near the ligament insertion site or through an external force transducer/force-moment sensor. Without confirming or denying the double-bundle theory of the ACL, it is biomechanically of interest to describe an anteromedial and posterolateral ligament portion as the cross-sectional dimension of the ACL has an anteromedial-posterolateral long axis and therefore, specific anteromedial and posterolateral biomechanical properties. In full extension, the in-situ force of the ACL as a response to anterior tibial translation of 143 N has been shown to be close to 100 N [16]. The PL bundle shows hereby a higher in-situ force compared to the AMB. In 15 degrees of flexion, the in-situ forces of the PLB and AMB both increase. With further flexion, the in-situ force of the PLB decreases significantly and drops beneath the in-situ force of the AMB, which slightly increases. These findings correlate with the assumption that the PLB lengthens in extension, while the AMB bundle lengthens in flexion. However, several studies have failed to reproduce these findings and show that the AMB carries a greater portion of the load at all flexion angles compared to the PLB, emphasising that the AM and PL bundle work synergistically rather than reciprocally. Central kinetic properties of ligaments comprise ultimate load to failure and linear stiffness, which has implications for reconstruction surgery and necessary graft properties. The ultimate load to failure of the ACL has been shown to be dependent on the age of the specimen. Younger specimens under the age of 35 years show an ultimate load of failure of 2,160 N, while older specimens over the age of 60 show an ultimate load to failure of 658 N [81]. Based on estimations, walking and descending stairs are thought to induce an ACL load of 169 and 445 N, respectively. The mean stiffness of the ACL has been measured to be 242 $\pm$ 28 N/mm in younger specimens and of 124 $\pm$ 16 N/mm in older specimens. There is still scientific debate regarding the lowest necessary ACL graft strength required for successful graft incorporation and stability. Numbers as low as 248 N have been found to be sufficient in the literature [90]. The tensile characteristics of a ligament may change depending on activity. Cyclic loading temporarily elongates the ACL and the resulting creep and relaxation have implications for the risk of ACL rupture.

# 3 Kinematics

The term kinematics describes the 3-dimensional geometry of a motion regarding displacement, acceleration and velocity. Forces are not considered. The assessment and description of knee kinematics represents a formidable challenge. Several imaging modalities have been used to chart in vivo and in vitro knee kinematics [26, 41, 61, 74, 80, 86]. However, a reliable measuring system to eliminate kinematic crosstalk and other potential misinterpretations of motions remains an experimental challenge. Knee kinematics are influenced by multiple factors including the geometry of the knee joint [19, 20, 56, 57, 84, 91, 99] and its supportive structures, ligament orientation and resistance, muscle-tension, rotation velocities of the hip and ankle joints, synovial fluid as well as inertia and damping. Knee joint kinematics are currently described based on 6 degrees of motional freedom, comprising 3 rotational movements (flexion and extension, internal and external rotation as well as varus and valgus angulation) and 3 translational movements (anterior and posterior glide, medial and lateral shift as well as compression and distraction). Translational movements are defined as rotational movements with the centre of rotation at infinity. The movement of flexion and extension represents a rotation around an axis perpendicular to the sagittal plane. A centre of rotation in this plane at infinity equates to translational movements in the form of anterior and posterior glide as well as compression and distraction. The movement of varus and valgus angulation represents a rotation around an axis perpendicular to the coronal plane. A centre of rotation in this plane at infinity equates to translational movements in the form of medial and lateral shift as well as compression and distraction. The movement of internal and external rotation represents a rotation around an axis perpendicular to the axial plane. A centre of rotation in this plane at infinity equates to translational movements in the form of medial and lateral shift as well as anterior and posterior glide. Pure translations, being the geometric transformation that moves every point of a figure the same distance in a given direction, are typically the result of external forces that overcome or parallelise the resistance of joint structures. In physiological knee kinematics, combined rotatory and translational movements are typically observed. The ratio of rotation and translation is dependent on resistance and rotational axes. The nature and function of rotational axes are still a matter of scientific debate. Theories of rotational axes propose models with instantaneous, fixed, helical as well as infinite axes [9]. The latter defines joint kinematics to be based on the geometry of joint surfaces and the length and resistance patterns of involved structures. The synergy of geometry and resistance is reflected in the association of knee flexion and femoro-tibial rotation. Even though flexion and extension are thought to occur based on poly-centric rotation, a fixed axis model has been introduced to facilitate the understanding of femoro-tibial contact areas [31]. The posterior femoral condyles are hereby thought to comprise two separate rotational axes which represent the radii of corresponding contact areas. The anterior-proximal axis represents the radius of a relatively large anterior contact area of the medial condyle and a relatively small contact area of the lateral condyle. The distal-posterior axis represents the radii of similar sized posterior contact areas of the medial and lateral posterior condyles. The medial tibial plateau comprises 4 zones and two slopes, while the lateral tibial plateau comprises 3 zones and 3 slopes. The anterior femoral contact areas articulate during extension. At approximately 15–20 degrees of flexion, the femur shifts to articulate through the posterior contact areas [31]. During flexion until 120°, the medial femoral condyle remains practically in situ, while the lateral condyle moves approximately 15 mm posteriorly towards the steeper posterior tibial slope. As the medial and lateral femoral condyles display different geometry but have the same rotational speed, knee flexion is associated with simultaneous rotation, which equates to internal tibial rotation/external femoral rotation. The concave medial tibial condyle supports rotation without significant translation while the flat lateral tibial condyle supports a combined rotatory and translational movement. The femoro-tibial rotation has also implications for patella tracking and patellar groove entry. From 120° to full flexion, both condyles shift posteriorly onto the posterior meniscal horn in order to create free space for full flexion, causing femoro-tibial joint subluxation. About 5 degrees of the rotation is undergone in the first 10 degrees of flexion, while a further 15 degrees of rotation occurs from 45 to 120°. Thus, the association of flexion/extension and rotation is not reserved to the screw home mechanism in terminal extension but occurs through full range of motion. The larger radius of the anterior lateral femoral contact area facilitates gliding in respect to rolling which is thought to have implications for non-contact ACL injury. The screw home mechanism is thought to be reversed by the popliteus muscle by inducing internal tibial rotation in full extension, hereby relaxing the tension of collateral ligaments for the inception of flexion [36]. The combined rotatory and translational movements of the femoral condyles can be expressed 2-dimensionally as the combination of rolling and sliding as proposed by Kaltenborn [6]. According to Kaltenborn, rolling and sliding represent rotatory movements on a circular path around specific rotation centres. In rolling, the rotation centre is located at the point of contact. In sliding, the rotation centre is located in the centre of the curvature. Isolated rolling movements of the femur imply substantial displacement and ultimately femoro-tibial luxation, which is thought to be prevented by a simultaneous sliding movement of the femur to maintain physiological joint alignment. The kinematic role of the ACL is not yet fully understood. Femoro-tibial rotatory control and the stabilisation of rotatory axes, especially when femoral contact areas are shifted, are thought to be fundamental functions of the ACL. Furthermore, the ACL is thought to resist anterior tibial translation near extension, where the flexion angle of the m. quadriceps has the worst mechanical advantage to extend the knee, inducing the greatest anterior directed force on the proximal tibia. Contra-intuitively, not only the quadriceps muscle but also hamstring muscles may be involved in knee extension based on the Lombard's paradox [48]. In vivo kinematic data suggest that the ACL primarily functions near full extension, based on the finding that the ACL consistently decreases in length throughout knee flexion. In the clinical setting, the pairing of forced anterior tibial translation and rotation is of interest. Coupled rotation describes the association of internal tibial rotation and anterior tibial translation. The exact mechanism is not yet fully understood. Differences in menisco-capsular attachments, condyle geometry, tethering mechanisms, friction and altering rotatory axes roam among potential reasons for the phenomenon. In the ACL intact knee, an anterior force applied to the tibia results in anterior tibial translation and internal rotation. The external force overcomes joint resistance, resulting in a primary translational movement. As the ACL and supporting structures are progressively tightened, the tibia is thought to be tethered and the centre of rotation is shifted towards the tibial ACL insertion site, hereby enhancing the rotatory nature of the movement. If the ACL is transected, the centre of rotation is thought to be shifted medially towards infinity, thereby enhancing the translatory nature of the movement. As a result, the resistance of collateral structures increases, reflected in the fact that the in-situ force of posterolateral ligamentous structures has been shown to increase by 413 percent [33] after the ACL is transected [33]. It has been hypothesised that the working principle of the ACL is not only to restrain internal rotation but to centralise the rotational axis in order to minimise cartilage and meniscal wear. In regard to the pivot-shift test, the importance of a 3-dimensional biomechanical model becomes obvious. Internal tibial torque in the ACL deficient knee near full extension leads to combined anterior tibial translation and internal tibial rotation. The translatory nature of the movement is enhanced as the centre of rotation is shifted medially based on ACL deficiency. As a result, the medial femoro-tibial contact area is brought forward and once the medial resistance increases, it becomes a new centre of rotation with a wider rotational path. Valgus stress stabilises the rotational axis and increases the uptake of potential energy. As the knee is flexed, the tibia is pulled back by the ITB relocating both the medial and lateral compartment. Even though controversially discussed, several authors have stated that ACL deficiency is mainly believed to be characterised by translation, not by rotation, and that ACL reconstructed knees tend to show increased laxity predominantly on translation and not on rotation. The synergy of peripheral and central structures of the knee is fundamental for normal knee kinematics. The overall function of ligaments depending on specific length patterns has been a central subject of joint biomechanics. In regard to the ACL, the fibre 's femoral attachment is thought to represent one of the most sensitive factors affecting length patterns during knee motion. The complexity of length-tension pattern of the ACL is thought to go beyond simplified descriptions of anteromedial fibres lengthening in knee flexion, and posterolateral fibres lengthening in knee extension. Based on the four-bar model by Menschik [59], Burmester mathematically determined corresponding isometric femoral and tibial locations of the knee joint. From the resulting cubic Burmester curve, isometric attachment sites around the knee joint may be derived [63]. The Burmester curve has limited clinical application as the shape of the curve depends on a specific knee flexion angle and is based on small infinitesimal knee motions. Isometric tibial attachment sites outside the curve have been determined when a wider range of knee motion is considered. However, the Burmester curve emphasises the synergy of central and peripheral joint stabilising structures based on their specific geometry. Several authors have reported that the Burmester curve may indicate isometric insertional points of LEAP. The fact that the embryonic ACL is functional before the final contouring of the condyles has given rise to the assumption that the geometry of the knee joint is influenced by ligamentous control.

## 4 ACL Failure Mechanism

The mechanism of ACL injury is not yet fully understood. Even though there is evidence for the biomechanical causality of several mechanisms [34, 45, 50, 53, 60, 71, 98], the in vivo influence of these mechanisms remains unknown. For instance, a cadaveric study found that aggressive musculus quadriceps contraction leads to anterior tibial translation [12]. The practical validity for the mechanism of ACL injury remains unknown based on unnaturally high forces used in the study. However, the hypothesis of the musculus quadriceps being involved in lowering the threshold force for ACL injury may be derived. The three-dimensional knee loads with the highest impact on ACL injury risk are the combination of muscular resistance to a large knee flexion moment, external reaction force inducing knee compression, internal tibial torque as well as knee abduction moment during a single leg manoeuvre [3]. While anterior tibial shear forces are thought to be the primary ACL loading mechanism, the influence and secondary order of importance concerning transverse and frontal plane ACL loading mechanisms remain unknown [3]. Even though cadaveric studies contribute to the biomechanical understanding of ACL injury, results have limited validity based on unphysiological testing conditions. In regard to video analysis, the time from ground contact to ACL injury may be shorter than the exposition time of a single frame of a video. As a result, the exact ACL injury mechanism is still unclear and different mechanisms and contributing factors regarding the aetiology of ACL injury are being discussed [54, 65, 72, 73, 77, 83, 84, 89, 91–94, 97, 99, 105, 107, 108]. In addition, recent evidence supports potential ACL failure through repetitive sub-maximal loading and accumulation of micro-damage in the ACL and supporting structures [21]. In general, a single "catastrophic" manoeuvre is typically assumed to induce ACL injury. ACL injuries are predominantly non-contact injuries [4, 5, 40, 93, 105, 107, 108]. It remains unclear at what time point the ACL is affected and if preceding mechanisms such as a relatively high knee flexion angle prior to the physiological coupled extension/rotation motion of the knee preparing ground contact are influential. ACL injury is currently believed to be the result of axial compressive forces at ground contact which induce a rotational knee movement based on specific and asymmetric tibio-femoral geometry. Muscular traction, knee abduction moment, relaxation and ligamentous creep may contribute to the mechanism of ACL injury. The direction and nature of tibio-femoral contact forces are dependent on several factors including body orientation and the degree of internal tibial rotation, femoro-tibial contact areas, slope and tilt [65]. Recently, the potentially overlooked effect of external tibial rotation on ACL injury susceptibility is being elucidated [83]. A combination of provocative joint-angle positions of the lower limb has been observed in non-contact ACL injuries comprising hip flexion, slight knee flexion and ankle extension [5]. It has been hypothesised that the combination of these joint positions may lower the threshold force needed for ACL injury. Heal landing is thought to accelerate the tibia anteriorly while abolishing absorbing properties of the calf muscles. The contribution of muscle activation to ACL injury remains unknown. Especially, the role of hamstring muscle contributing to knee extension based on Lombard's paradox remains unclear. Specific bone bruise patterns from tibio-femoral collision are typically seen following ACL injury. However, there is conflicting evidence about the genesis. The femur may collide with the posterior aspect of the tibia while being forced into extension as described in the hip-flexion-knee-extension paradox [24], or during a repositioning manoeuvre in flexion following femoro-tibial subluxation. As several studies find no rotational or valgus moment under ACL injury, it remains unclear to what extent tibial rotation and valgus moment represent risk factors of ACL injury or are part of a collapsing event following ACL injury. The susceptibility of ACL injury has been shown to be influenced by several biomechanical factors [29, 30, 58, 75, 78, 106, 107, 112]. Among geometrical factors roam tibial bony slope, slope asymmetry, tibial cartilage slope, meniscal slope, ACL volume, femoral notch width, concavity depth of the medial tibial condyle, femoral condyle geometry, patella related mechanisms as well as meniscal bone angle. In general, geometrical factors that modulate the nature and velocity of femoro-tibial rotation under compressive forces are thought to contribute to the mechanism of ACL injury [84].

## References


1. Ahmed AM, McLean C. In vitro measurement of the restraining role of the anterior cruciate ligament during walking and stair ascent. J Biomech Eng. 2002;124.
2. Banovetz MT, Kennedy NI, LaPrade RF, Engebretsen L, Moatshe G. Biomechanical considerations for graft choice in anterior cruciate ligament reconstruction. Ann Joint. 2023;8.
3. Beaulieu M, Ashton-Miller J, Wojtys E. Loading mechanisms of the anterior cruciate ligament. Sports Biomech. 2021;22:1–29.
4. Boden BP, Dean GS, Feagin JA, Garrett WE. Mechanisms of anterior cruciate ligament injury. Orthopedics. 2000;23.
5. Boden BP, Sheehan FT, Torg JS, Hewett TE. Noncontact anterior cruciate ligament injuries: mechanisms and risk factors. J Am Acad Orthop Surg. 2010;18(9):520–7.
6. Brandt C, Sole G, Krause MW, Nel M. An evidence-based review on the validity of the Kaltenborn rule as applied to the glenohumeral joint. Man Ther. 2007;12(1):3–11.
7. Butler DL, Noyes FR, Grood ES. Ligamentous restraints to anterior-posterior drawer in the human knee. A biomechanical study. J Bone Joint Surg Am. 1980;62.
8. Cabuk H, Kusku Cabuk F. Mechanoreceptors of the ligaments and tendons around the knee. Clin Anat. 2016;29.
9. Christopher DS, Jones PN. The biomechanics of the anterior cruciate ligament and its reconstruction (Internet). In: Theoretical Biomechanics. InTech; 2011. Available from: https://doi.org/10.5772/19939
10. Coobs BR, Wijdicks CA, Armitage BM, Spiridonov SI, Westerhaus BD, Johansen S. An in vitro analysis of an anatomical medial knee reconstruction. Am J Sports Med. 2010;38.
11. Dargel J, Gotter M, Mader K, Pennig D, Koebke J, Schmidt-Wiethoff R. Biomechanics of the anterior cruciate ligament and implications for surgical reconstruction. Strategies Trauma Limb Reconstr. 2007;2(1):1–12.
12. DeMorat G, Weinhold P, Blackburn T, Chudik S, Garrett W. Aggressive quadriceps loading can induce noncontact anterior cruciate ligament injury. Am J Sports Med. 2004;32.
13. Domnick C, Raschke MJ, Herbort M. Biomechanics of the anterior cruciate ligament: physiology, rupture and reconstruction techniques. World J Orthop. 2016;7(2):82–93.
14. Fleming BC, Beynnon BD, Tohyama H, Johnson RJ, Nichols CE, Renstrom P. Determination of a zero strain reference for the anteromedial band of the anterior cruciate ligament. J Orthop Res: Off Publ Orthop Res Soc. 1994;12.
15. Fleming BC, Renstrom PA, Beynnon BD, Engstrom B, Peura GD, Badger GJ, et al. The effect of weightbearing and external loading on anterior cruciate ligament strain. J Biomech. 2001;34.
16. Fu FH, Bennett CH, Lattermann C, Ma CB. Current trends in anterior cruciate ligament reconstruction. Part 1: Biology and biomechanics of reconstruction. Am J Sports Med. 1999 Nov-Dec;27(6):821–30. https://doi.org/10.1177/03635465990270062501. PMID: 10569374.
17. Fukubayashi T, Torzilli PA, Sherman MF, Warren RF. An in vitro biomechanical evaluation of anterior-posterior motion of the knee. Tibial displacement, rotation, and torque. J Bone Jt Surg Am. 1982;64.
18. Gardner EJ, Noyes FR, Jetter AW, Grood ES, Harms SP, Levy MS. Effect of anteromedial and posterolateral anterior cruciate ligament bundles on resisting medial and lateral tibiofemoral compartment subluxations. Arthroscopy. 2015;31.
19. Giffin JR. Effects of increasing tibial slope on the biomechanics of the knee. Am J Sports Med. 2004;32.

20. Giffin JR, Vogrin TM, Zantop T, Woo SL, Harner CD. Effects of increasing tibial slope on the biomechanics of the knee. Am J Sports Med. 2004;32.
21. Grodman LH, Beaulieu ML, Ashton-Miller JA, Wojtys EM. Levels of ACL-straining activities increased in the six months prior to non-contact ACL injury in a retrospective survey: evidence consistent with ACL fatigue failure. Front Physiol. 2023;14:1166980.
22. Guenoun D, Vaccaro J, Corroller T, Barral PA, Lagier A, Pauly V, et al. A dynamic study of the anterior cruciate ligament of the knee using an open MRI. Surg Radiol Anat. 2017;39.
23. Harms SP, Noyes FR, Grood ES, Jetter AW, Huser LE, Levy MS, et al. Anatomic single-graft anterior cruciate ligament reconstruction restores rotational stability: a robotic study in cadaveric knees. Arthroscopy. 2015;31.
24. Hashemi J, Breighner R, Chandrashekar N, Hardy DM, Chaudhari AM, Shultz SJ, et al. Hip extension, knee flexion paradox: a new mechanism for non-contact ACL injury. J Biomech. 2011;44.
25. Hefzy MS, Grood ES, Noyes FR. Factors affecting the region of most isometric femoral attachments. Part II: the anterior cruciate ligament. Am J Sports Med. 1989;17.
26. Hemmerich A, van der Merwe W, Vaughan CL. Measuring three-dimensional knee kinematics under torsional loading. J Biomech. 2009;42(2):183–6.
27. Hewett TE, Ford KR, Hoogenboom BJ, Myer GD. Understanding and preventing acl injuries: current biomechanical and epidemiologic considerations—update 2010. N Am J Sports Phys Ther. 2010;5.
28. Hewett TE, Ford KR, Xu YY, Khoury J, Myer GD. Utilization of ACL injury biomechanical and neuromuscular risk profile analysis to determine the effectiveness of neuromuscular training. Am J Sports Med. 2016;44.
29. Hodel S, Postolka B, Flury A, Schütz P, Taylor W, Vlachopoulos L, et al. Influence of bone morphology on in vivo tibio-femoral kinematics in healthy knees during gait activities. J Clin Med. 2022;11:5082.
30. Imran A, O'Connor JJ. Theoretical estimates of cruciate ligament forces: effects of tibial surface geometry and ligament orientations. Proc Inst Mech Eng H. 1997;211.
31. Iwaki H, Pinskerova V, Freeman MA. Tibiofemoral movement 1: the shapes and relative movements of the femur and tibia in the unloaded cadaver knee. J Bone Joint Surg Br. 2000;82(8):1189–95.
32. Kakarlapudi TK, Bickerstaff DR. Knee instability—isolated and complex. West J Med. 2001;174.
33. Kanamori A, Sakane M, Zeminski J, Rudy TW, Woo SL. In-situ force in the medial and lateral structures of intact and ACL-deficient knees. J Orthop Sci. 2000;5(6):567–71.
34. Kanamori A, Zeminski J, Rudy TW, Li G, Fu FH, Woo SL. The effect of axial tibial torque on the function of the anterior cruciate ligament: a biomechanical study of a simulated pivot shift test. Arthrosc: J Arthrosc Relat Surg: Off Publ Arthrosc Assoc North Am Int Arthrosc Assoc. 2002;18.
35. Kiapour AM, Quatman CE, Goel VK, Wordeman SC, Hewett TE, Demetropoulos CK. Timing sequence of multi-planar knee kinematics revealed by physiologic cadaveric simulation of landing: implications for ACL injury mechanism. Clin Biomech (Bristol, Avon). 2014;29.
36. Kim D, Asai S, Moon CW, Hwang SC, Lee S, Keklikci K. Biomechanical evaluation of anatomic single- and double-bundle anterior cruciate ligament reconstruction techniques using the quadriceps tendon. Knee Surg Sports Traumatol Arthrosc. 2015;23.
37. Kim HY, Kim KJ, Yang DS, Jeung SW, Choi HG, Choy WS. Screw-home movement of the tibiofemoral joint during normal gait: three-dimensional analysis. Clin Orthop Surg. 2015;7(3):303–9.
38. Kim YK, Yoo JD, Kim SW, Park SH, Cho JH, Lim HM. Intraoperative graft isometry in anatomic single-bundle anterior cruciate ligament reconstruction. Knee Surg Relat Res. 2018;30.
39. Kocher MS, Steadman JR, Briggs KK, Sterett WI, Hawkins RJ. Relationships between objective assessment of ligament stability and subjective assessment of symptoms and function after anterior cruciate ligament reconstruction. Am J Sports Med. 2004;32.

40. Koga H, Nakamae A, Shima Y, Iwasa J, Myklebust G, Engebretsen L, et al. Mechanisms for noncontact anterior cruciate ligament injuries: knee joint kinematics in 10 injury situations from female team handball and basketball. Am J Sports Med. 2010;38.
41. Krosshaug T, Nakamae A, Boden B, Engebretsen L, Smith G, Slauterbeck J, et al. Estimating 3D joint kinematics from video sequences of running and cutting maneuvers—assessing the accuracy of simple visual inspection. Gait Posture. 2007;26.
42. Lee H, Petrofsky JS, Daher N, Berk L, Laymon M, Khowailed IA. Anterior cruciate ligament elasticity and force for flexion during the menstrual cycle. Med Sci Monit. 2013;19.
43. Lentz TA, Zeppieri G, George SZ, Tillman SM, Moser MW, Farmer KW, et al. Comparison of physical impairment, functional, and psychosocial measures based on fear of reinjury/lack of confidence and return-to-sport status after ACL reconstruction. Am J Sports Med. 2015;43.
44. Levy IM, Torzilli PA, Gould JD, Warren RF. The effect of lateral meniscectomy on motion of the knee. J Bone Jt Surg Am. 1989;71.
45. Li G, Rudy TW, Sakane M, Kanamori A, Ma CB, Woo SL. The importance of quadriceps and hamstring muscle loading on knee kinematics and in-situ forces in the ACL. J Biomech. 1999;32.
46. Lipke JM, Janecki CJ, Nelson CL, McLeod P, Thompson C, Thompson J. The role of incompetence of the anterior cruciate and lateral ligaments in anterolateral and anteromedial instability. A biomechanical study of cadaver knees. J Bone Joint Surg Am Vol. 1981;63.
47. Livesay GA, Fujie H, Kashiwaguchi S, Morrow DA, Fu FH, Woo SL. Determination of the in situ forces and force distribution within the human anterior cruciate ligament. Ann Biomed Eng. 1995;23(4):467–74.
48. Lombard WP, Abbott FM. The mechanical effects produced by the contraction of individual muscles of the thigh of the frog. Am J Physiol. 1907;20:1–60.
49. Lopomo N, Zaffagnini S, Bignozzi S, Visani A, Marcacci M. Pivot-shift test: analysis and quantification of knee laxity parameters using a navigation system. J Orthop Res. 2010;28(2):164–9.
50. MacWilliams BA, Wilson DR, DesJardins JD, Romero J, Chao EY. Hamstrings cocontraction reduces internal rotation, anterior translation, and anterior cruciate ligament load in weight-bearing flexion. J Orthop Res. 1999;17.
51. Mancini EJ, Kohen R, Esquivel AO, Cracchiolo AM, Lemos SE. Comparison of ACL strain in the MCL-Deficient and MCL-reconstructed knee during simulated landing in a cadaveric model. Am J Sports Med. 2017;45.
52. Marieswaran M, Jain I, Garg B, Sharma V, Kalyanasundaram D. A review on biomechanics of anterior cruciate ligament and materials for reconstruction. Appl Bionics Biomech. 2018;2018:4657824.
53. Markolf KL, Bargar WL, Shoemaker SC, Amstutz HC. The role of joint load in knee stability. J Bone Jt Surg Am. 1981;63.
54. Markolf KL, Burchfield DM, Shapiro MM, Shepard MF, Finerman GA, Slauterbeck JL. Combined knee loading states that generate high anterior cruciate ligament forces. J Orthop Res. 1995;13.
55. Markolf KL, Willems MJ, Jackson SR, Finerman GA. In situ calibration of miniature sensors implanted into the anterior cruciate ligament part II: force probe measurements. J Orthop Res: Off Publ Orthop Res Soc. 1998;16.
56. Marouane H, Shirazi-Adl A, Hashemi J. Quantification of the role of tibial posterior slope in knee joint mechanics and ACL force in simulated gait. J Biomech. 2015;48.
57. Matsuda S, Miura H, Nagamine R, Urabe K, Ikenoue T, Okazaki K, et al. Posterior tibial slope in the normal and varus knee. Am J Knee Surg. 1999;12.
58. McLean SG, Oh YK, Palmer ML, Lucey SM, Lucarelli DG, Ashton-Miller JA. The relationship between anterior tibial acceleration, tibial slope, and ACL strain during a simulated jump landing task. J Bone Jt Surg Am. 2011;93.
59. Menschik A. Mechanik des Kniegelenkes. 1 [Mechanics of the knee-joint. 1 (author's transl)]. Z Orthop Ihre Grenzgeb. 1974 Jun;112(3):481–95. German. PMID: 4277228.

60. Meyer EG, Haut RC. Excessive compression of the human tibio-femoral joint causes ACL rupture. J Biomech. 2005;38.
61. Monaco E, Ferretti A, Labianca L, Maestri B, Speranza A, Kelly MJ. Navigated knee kinematics after cutting of the ACL and its secondary restraint. Knee Surg, Sports Traumatol, Arthrosc: Off J ESSKA. 2012;20.
62. More RC, Karras BT, Neiman F, Fritschy D, Woo SLY, Daniel DM. Hamstrings-an anterior cruciate ligament protagonist: an in vitro study. Am J Sports Med. 1993;21.
63. Müller W, Telger TC. The Knee: Form, Function, and Ligament Reconstruction: Springer-Verlag; 1983.
64. Myer GD, Ford KR, Khoury J, Succop P, Hewett TE. Biomechanics laboratory-based prediction algorithm to identify female athletes with high knee loads that increase risk of ACL injury. Br J Sports Med. 2011;45.
65. Navacchia A, Bates NA, Schilaty ND, Krych AJ, Hewett TE. Knee abduction and internal rotation moments increase ACL force during landing through the posterior slope of the tibia. J Orthop Res. 2019;37(8):1730–42.
66. Nawabi D, Imhauser C, Tucker S, Nguyen J, Wickiewicz T, Pearle A. ACL fibers inserting on the lateral intercondylar ridge carry the greatest loads—are modern anatomic femoral tunnel positions too low? Orthopaed J Sports Med. 2014;2.
67. Noyes FR, Grood ES. The scientific basis for examination and classification of knee ligament injuries. Noyes' knee disorders: surgery, rehabilitation, clinical outcomes. Philadelphia: Elsevier; 2017.
68. Noyes FR, Grood ES, Butler DL, Malek M. Clinical laxity tests and functional stability of the knee: biomechanical concepts. Clin Orthop Relat Res. 1980;146.
69. Noyes FR, Grood ES, Torzilli PA. Current concepts review. The definitions of terms for motion and position of the knee and injuries of the ligaments. J Bone Joint Surg Am. 1989;71.
70. Noyes FR, Jetter AW, Grood ES, Harms SP, Gardner EJ, Levy MS. Anterior cruciate ligament function in providing rotational stability assessed by medial and lateral tibiofemoral compartment translations and subluxations. Am J Sports Med. 2015;43.
71. Oh YK, Kreinbrink JL, Wojtys EM, Ashton-Miller JA. Effect of axial tibial torque direction on ACL relative strain and strain rate in an in vitro simulated pivot landing. J Orthop Res. 2012;30.
72. Oh YK, Lipps DB, Ashton-Miller JA, Wojtys EM. What strains the anterior cruciate ligament during a pivot landing? Am J Sports Med. 2012;40.
73. Pandy MG, Shelburne KB. Dependence of cruciate-ligament loading on muscle forces and external load. J Biomech. 1997;30.
74. Papannagari R, Gill TJ, Defrate LE, Moses JM, Petruska AJ, Li G. In vivo kinematics of the knee after anterior cruciate ligament reconstruction: a clinical and functional evaluation. Am J Sports Med. 2006;34.
75. Pappas E, Shiyko MP, Ford KR, Myer GD, Hewett TE. Biomechanical deficit profiles associated with ACL injury risk in female athletes. Med Sci Sports Exerc. 2016;48.
76. Park J-G, Han S-B, Lee C-S, Jeon O, Jang K-M. Anatomy, biomechanics, and reconstruction of the anterolateral ligament of the knee joint. Medicina. 2022;58:786.
77. Pollard CD, Sigward SM, Powers CM. Limited hip and knee flexion during landing is associated with increased frontal plane knee motion and moments. Clin Biomech (Bristol, Avon). 2010;25.
78. Renstrom P, Arms SW, Stanwyck TS, Johnson RJ, Pope MH. Strain within the anterior cruciate ligament during hamstring and quadriceps activity. Am J Sports Med. 1986;14.
79. Robinson JR, Bull AM, Amis AA. Structural properties of the medial collateral ligament complex of the human knee. J Biomech. 2005;38.
80. Rudy TW, Livesay GA, Woo SL, Fu FH. A combined robotic/universal force sensor approach to determine in situ forces of knee ligaments. J Biomech. 1996;29.
81. Runer A, Keeling L, Wagala N, Nugraha H, Özbek EA, Hughes JD, et al. Current trends in graft choice for anterior cruciate ligament reconstruction—part I: anatomy, biomechanics, graft incorporation and fixation. J Exp Orthop. 2023;10(1):37.

82. Sakane M, Fox RJ, Woo SL, Livesay GA, Li G, Fu FH. In situ forces in the anterior cruciate ligament and its bundles in response to anterior tibial loads. J Orthop Res. 1997;15(2):285–93.
83. Santos CF, Bastos R, Andrade R, Pereira R, Parente MPL, Jorge RN, et al. Revisiting the role of knee external rotation in non-contact ACL mechanism of injury. Appl Sci. 2023;13(6):3802.
84. Sauer S, Clatworthy M. Editorial commentary: the ratio of tibial slope and meniscal bone angle is a strong predictor for anterior cruciate ligament injury: a steep hill and a shallow speed bump are a hazardous combination. Arthroscopy. 2021;37(5):1610–1.
85. Scanlan SF, Chaudhari AM, Dyrby CO, Andriacchi TP. Differences in tibial rotation during walking in ACL reconstructed and healthy contralateral knees. J Biomech. 2010;43.
86. Scarvell J, Smith P, Refshauge K, Galloway H, Woods K. Comparison of kinematic analysis by mapping tibiofemoral contact with movement of the femoral condylar centres in healthy and anterior cruciate ligament injured knees. J Orthopaed Res Off Publ Orthopaed Res Soc. 2004;22:955–62.
87. Serack F, Holwell N, Amsden BG. Polymer scaffolds for anterior cruciate ligament tissue engineering. Functional biopolymers. Cham: Springer International Publishing; 2018. p. 1–30.
88. Shao Q, MacLeod TD, Manal K, Buchanan TS. Estimation of ligament loading and anterior tibial translation in healthy and ACL-deficient knees during gait and the influence of increasing tibial slope using EMG-driven approach. Ann Biomed Eng. 2011;39.
89. Sheehan FT, Sipprell WH, Boden BP. Dynamic sagittal plane trunk control during anterior cruciate ligament injury. Am J Sports Med. 2012;40.
90. Shelbourne KD, Gray T. Anterior cruciate ligament reconstruction with autogenous patellar tendon graft followed by accelerated rehabilitation. A two- to nine-year followup. Am J Sports Med. 1997;25(6):786–95.
91. Shelburne KB, Kim HJ, Sterett WI, Pandy MG. Effect of posterior tibial slope on knee biomechanics during functional activity. J Orthop Res. 2011;29.
92. Shelburne KB, Torry MR, Pandy MG. Contributions of muscles, ligaments, and the ground-reaction force to tibiofemoral joint loading during normal gait. J Orthop Res. 2006;24.
93. Shimokochi Y, Shultz SJ. Mechanisms of noncontact anterior cruciate ligament injury. J Athl Train. 2008;43.
94. Shin CS, Chaudhari AM, Andriacchi TP. Valgus plus internal rotation moments increase anterior cruciate ligament strain more than either alone. Med Sci Sports Exerc. 2011;43.
95. Shino K, Nakata K, Nakamura N, Toritsuka Y, Horibe S, Nakagawa S, et al. Rectangular tunnel double-bundle anterior cruciate ligament reconstruction with bone–patellar tendon–bone graft to mimic natural fiber arrangement. Arthroscopy. 2008;24.
96. Sidles JA, Larson RV, Garbini JL, Downey DJ, Matsen FA. Ligament length relationship in the moving knee. J Orthop Res. 1988;6.
97. Siegel L, Vandenakker-Albanese C, Siegel D. Anterior cruciate ligament injuries: anatomy, physiology, biomechanics, and management. Clin J Sport Med: Off J Can Acad Sport Med. 2012;22:349–55.
98. Solomonow M, Baratta R, Zhou BH, Shoji H, Bose W, Beck C, et al. The synergistic action of the anterior cruciate ligament and thigh muscles in maintaining joint stability. Am J Sports Med. 1987;15.
99. Stijak L, Herzog RF, Schai P. Is there an influence of the tibial slope of the lateral condyle on the ACL lesion? A case-control study. Knee Surg Sports Traumatol Arthrosc. 2008;16.
100. Swedberg AM, Reese SP, Maas SA, Ellis BJ, Weiss JA. Continuum description of the Poisson's ratio of ligament and tendon under finite deformation. J Biomech. 2014;47(12):3201–9.
101. Takatsu T, Itokazu M, Shimizu K, Brown TD. The function of posterior tilt of the tibial component following posterior cruciate ligament-retaining total knee arthroplasty. Bull Hosp Jt Dis. 1998;57.
102. Terauchi M, Hatayama K, Yanagisawa S, Saito K, Takagishi K. Sagittal alignment of the knee and Its relationship to noncontact anterior cruciate ligament injuries. Am J Sports Med. 2011;39.
103. Todd MS, Lalliss S, Garcia E, DeBerardino TM, Cameron KL. The relationship between posterior tibial slope and anterior cruciate ligament injuries. Am J Sports Med. 2010;38.

104. Torzilli PA, Deng X, Warren RF. The effect of joint-compressive load and quadriceps muscle force on knee motion in the intact and anterior cruciate ligament-sectioned knee. Am J Sports Med. 1994;22.
105. Uhorchak JM, Scoville CR, Williams GN, Arciero RA, St Pierre P, Taylor DC. Risk factors associated with noncontact injury of the anterior cruciate ligament: a prospective four-year evaluation of 859 West Point cadets. Am J Sports Med. 2003;31.
106. Voos JE, Suero EM, Citak M, Petrigliano FP, Bosscher MR, Wickiewicz TL, et al. Effect of tibial slope on the stability of the anterior cruciate ligament-deficient knee. Knee Surg Sports Traumatol Arthrosc. 2011.
107. Walden M, Krosshaug T, Bjorneboe J, Andersen TE, Faul O, Hagglund M. Three distinct mechanisms predominate in non-contact anterior cruciate ligament injuries in male professional football players: a systematic video analysis of 39 cases. Br J Sports Med. 2015;49.
108. Wall SJ, Rose DM, Sutter EG, Belkoff SM, Boden BP. The role of axial compressive and quadriceps forces in noncontact anterior cruciate ligament injury: a cadaveric study. Am J Sports Med. 2011.
109. Wang J-H, Li K, O'Farrell M, Harner C, Zhang X. Tension Pattern of the Cruciate Ligament Fibers During Rolling and Sliding; 2009.
110. Weber W, Weber EF. Mechanik der menschlichen Gehwerkzeuge: Eine anatomisch-physiologische Untersuchung. Göttingen: Dieterich; 1836–1836.
111. Wells HC, Sizeland KH, Kayed HR, Kirby N, Hawley A, Mudie ST, et al. Poisson's ratio of collagen fibrils measured by small angle X-ray scattering of strained bovine pericardium. J Appl Phys. 2015;117(4).
112. Whitney DC, Sturnick DR, Vacek PM, DeSarno MJ, Gardner-Morse M, Tourville TW, et al. Relationship between the risk of suffering a first-time noncontact ACL injury and geometry of the femoral notch and ACL: a prospective cohort study with a nested case-control analysis. Am J Sports Med. 2014;42.
113. Willinger L, Athwal K, Holthof S, Imhoff A, Williams A, Amis A. Role of the Anterior Cruciate Ligament, anterolateral complex, and lateral meniscus posterior root in anterolateral rotatory knee instability: a biomechanical study. Am J Sports Med. 2023;51:036354652311610.
114. Woo SLY, Hollis JM, Adams DJ, Lyon RM, Takai S. Tensile properties of the human femur-anterior cruciate ligament-tibia complex. The effects of specimen age and orientation. Am J Sports Med. 1991;19.
115. Yang S, Liu Y, Ma S, Ding C, Kong Z, Li H, et al. Stress and strain changes of the anterior cruciate ligament at different knee flexion angles: A three-dimensional finite element study. J Orthop Sci. 2023.
116. Zhang Z-y, Pan NX, Maimaitijiang P, Meng L-y, He Z-y, Zhao Q, et al. Anterior tibial subluxation measured under a modified protocol is positively correlated with posterior tibial slope: a comparative study of MRI measurement methods. Knee Surg Sports Traumatol Arthrosc. 2022;30.
117. Zhou T, Xu Y, Zhou L, Wang S, Wang S, Xu W. Multi-planar instability, laxity and reduced knee flexion during the support phase of walking are determinants of return to sports. Front Bioeng Biotechnol. 2022;10.

# ACL Reconstruction

## 1 Introduction

ACL reconstruction represents the gold standard in the treatment of symptomatic ACL insufficiency based on improved stability and reduced risk of consecutive cartilage and meniscus injury when compared to non-operative treatment. However, ACL reconstruction is currently not consistently superior to non-operative treatment in terms of subjective outcomes, long term activity level or risk of OA development [137]. ACLR is indicated for patients of all age groups with significant knee instability who intend to return to a relevant level of sports rather than a change in lifestyle [18, 26]. Graft implantation improves knee stability and serves as the structural foundation for the ligamentization process. As ACL deficiency is associated with altered kinematics, structural changes of the knee including alteration of cartilage slopes shortly after ACL injury may be observed. In addition, current ACL reconstruction techniques do not restore or regenerate native ACL properties including the force-attuning multilayered anchor architecture of the ACL. As a result, native biomechanics are typically not restored following ACL reconstruction and even though a central rotatory axis is re-established, residual dynamic rotatory laxity clinically manifested by a positive pivot-shift test, is increasingly recognised as a common finding following ACL reconstruction. In synergy with ongoing improvement of the anatomic and functional understanding of the ACL, surgical ACL reconstruction techniques have constantly been refined in accordance with reliable hardware and sophisticated technology [20, 135]. However, the ongoing endeavour for ultimate improvement of ACLR outcomes seems to continue. Several fundamental aspects of ACLR including timing, graft choice, tunnel placement, graft fixation technique as well as the management of concomitant pathology and indication of concomitant procedures are controversially discussed based on insufficient or conflicting evidence.

 
S. Sauer, *ACL Reconstruction: Current Concepts*,
https://doi.org/10.1007/978-3-031-69000-6_3

# 2 Diagnostics

## 2.1 *Anamnesis*

Detailed descriptions of present and previous injury episodes as well as resulting acute and chronic symptomatology are typically recorded. Important features that are associated with specific injury patterns include the nature, geometry and velocity of the injury motion. Contact injuries are associated with higher incidence and complexity of concomitant injuries. However, following non-contact ACL injury, concomitant meniscal and/or ligamentous pathology is easily overlooked. Low velocity injuries have been shown to be more frequently associated with bony avulsions including spine avulsions in the juvenile population. Among patient reported ACL injury mechanisms roam pivoting manoeuvres, rotational movements as well as hyper-extensional knee excursions. The majority of ACL injuries occurs through non-contact traumas [14, 16, 76], especially in deceleration or landing manoeuvres with the lower extremity in injury-provocative positions, comprising hip flexion, slight knee flexion and a planted foot [15]. Ground reaction force is hereby thought to bypass the normally absorption-competent triceps surae group, exerting unrestrained compressive forces on the femoro-tibial contact area. An audible pop is typically noted and has been shown to be associated with a positive predictive value of 100% regarding ACL injury in the juvenile population [31]. In addition to the injury mechanism, present and previous symptoms are recorded. Acutely, hemarthrosis, pain and instability resulting in incapability of resuming activity are usually present. The presence of hemarthrosis has been shown to be associated with ACL injury in over 70% of the cases. The gait cycle and terminal ROM are usually compromised. Chronically, muscle weakness and/or muscle atrophy, ROM deficits or pain in terminal ROM, catching and locking, subtle alterations of the gait cycle and instability with or without giving way phenomenon are typically reported. The subjective impression of unrestrained hyperextension is commonly reported. Information regarding previous ipsi and contralateral limb pathology, treatment procedures but also level of function, profession, and any information that has impact on treatment strategies is assessed. Psychological factors and the necessity of ACLR are discussed.

## 2.2 *Physical Examination*

Physical examination of patients with potential ACL injury comprises inspection, palpation, ROM assessment and specific tests including assessment of ligamentous integrity. The examination intends not only to recognise a possible injury but also to evaluate its complexity and resulting impact. In the acute setting, physical examination typically intends to assess for any pathology that needs further evaluation. In the non-acute setting, especially if the diagnosis has been established by means of MRI, physical examination intends to establish clinical associations and elaborate possible treatment strategies. In the non-acute setting, physical examination typically commences with the inspection of the gait cycle. Signs of instability such as fear of loading and limping may be revealed. Gait abnormalities such as a thrust gait may indicate collateral ligament injury. Inspection of the knee may reveal effusion and periarticular swelling around the knee, indicating potential intra and extra-articular injury. In chronic cases, muscle atrophy is commonly seen. Cicatrises from previous surgical procedures are assessed and reported with implications for further treatment strategies. The assessment of muscle appearance indicates level of function. When palpating the knee, excessive swelling is obvious. In chronic cases, only a subtle suprapatellar fluctuation sign may be present. Palpation of specific areas of the knee is performed to assess possible concomitant ligamentous, capsular, bony or cartilage injury. Tenderness along the joint line as well as a reproducible pop sensation may be associated with underlying meniscal pathology. Baker cysts indicate chronic effusion and synovitis. Assessment of range of motion intends to detect concomitant injuries and the neuromuscular condition of the knee which has implications for ACLR timing. Hyperextension of the uninjured leg should be assessed and recorded as hyperextension over 5 degrees has been found to be an independent risk factor of ACLR failure [49, 160]. Extension deficits may indicate displaced meniscal injuries. Severely compromised preoperative ROM is thought to be associated with higher incidence of postoperative complications. Several tests are used to assess ACL integrity including the Lachman test, the anterior drawer test and the pivot-shift test. The Lachman test compares the extent of femoro-tibial displacement between the injured and uninjured knee. In 15–30 degrees of flexion, the tibia is pulled forward to assess the amount of femoro-tibial displacement and nature of the resulting endpoint. The side-to-side difference, measured in millimetres, corresponds to ACL integrity and is classified into different grades of laxity. 1–2 mm side-to-side difference is regarded as normal. 3–5 mm side-to-side difference is defined as mild laxity. 6–10 mm is defined as moderate laxity. More than 10 mm side-to-side difference is defined as severe laxity. Even though the Lachman test is substantially dependent on several factors including PCL integrity, concomitant bucket handle meniscus lesion, the physician's technique and hand size as well as the degree of patient relaxation, a sensitivity of over 90% is typically described in the literature, succeeding the sensitivity of the anterior drawer test. For the latter, the patient is positioned supine with the knee in 90 degrees of flexion. Allowing the lower leg to hang freely is thought to minimise potential sources of error. The lower leg is then pulled forward and the extent of the possible femoro-tibial displacement, along with the quality of the endpoint is assessed. The anterior drawer test has been reported to indicate ACL injury, if the lower leg can be displaced more than 0.5 cm. The pivot-shift test is regarded as the most important test for assessment of ACL injury as it takes rotational instability into account [61, 62, 77, 88, 89, 98, 110]. With the patient lying supine, the knee is extended, the tibia is internally rotated, and a valgus load is applied. The lateral femoro-tibial compartment is thereby subluxed due to ACL deficiency. Once the traction vector of the IT-band becomes posteriorly directed in higher flexion angles, the lateral femorotibial joint is reduced [98]. The reduction-motion is categorised into three grades according to the corresponding sensory perception.

Grade I represents a subtle glide, grade II represents a more evident glide and grade III a gross glide. A more evident positive pivot-shift test is typically associated with concomitant pathology. The pivot-shift test requires an intact MCL. Increased tibial slope has been found to be associated with a more distinct pivot-shift movement. The reliability of all of the aforementioned tests has been questioned when performed in the conscious patient and clinical examination alone is rarely used to definitively diagnose ACL injury. However, it provides valuable information for further evaluation and preoperative planning. MRI is typically performed to confirm the diagnosis and assess the extent and complexity of the injury. The assessment of other ligamentous structures of the knee including MCL, LCL, PCL, PLC is strongly recommended as overlooked concomitant ligamentous pathology is associated with higher ACLR failure rate. A comprehensive evaluation, including patient history, physical examination, and appropriate imaging are thought to be of paramount importance for the diagnosis and treatment of knee injuries that involve ACL injury [31].

## 2.3 *Imaging*

MRI represents the gold standard for the diagnosis of ACL injury with accuracy, sensitivity and specificity of over 90%. In addition, partial injuries can typically be distinguished from complete tears, even though the functionality of the remaining tissue needs to be clinically verified. ACL tear location as well as concomitant injuries can be identified. For graft harvest, hamstring tendon dimension for the estimation of final graft volume can be assessed. For grafts involving patellar bone blocks, patella hypoplasia (being a contraindication for bone-block harvest) can be ruled out. Complete tears with reattachment of vital ACL stumps to the synovial envelope of the PCL as well as bridging tears with extensive reparative fibrosis represent a diagnostic challenge. 3 T imaging, oblique planes and flexion imaging have been found to enhance diagnostic accuracy. MRI findings can be divided into direct and indirect signs. Direct signs include ACL discontinuity, thickening and edema, abnormal signal and orientation as well as an empty notch sign on coronal sequences. Indirect signs include bone bruising of the lateral femoral condyle and tibial plateau [106], over 6 mm of anterior tibial translation, uncovered posterior horn of the lateral meniscus, Segond fracture, arcuate sign, PCL relaxation, collateral ligament injury, coronal lateral collateral ligament sign as well as a lateral femoral sulcus deeper than 1.5 mm. Bone bruising and a deep lateral femoral notch sign are strong indicators of ACL injury but not pathognomonic, especially in juvenile patients with increased ACL fibre elasticity. The Bosch-Bock bump (healed Segond fracture) typically indicates chronic ACL deficiency. Increased femoro-tibial displacement is commonly seen in knee extension in the lateral compartment. Severe rotational misalignment is indicative of combined ACL and ALC injury and results commonly in the visualisation of the entire PCL and LCL on a single coronal slice [116]. Partial tears show a combination of increased signal and fibre laxity. A gap sign (a gap between the lateral femoral condyle and the ACL) or a footprint sign (incomplete insertional

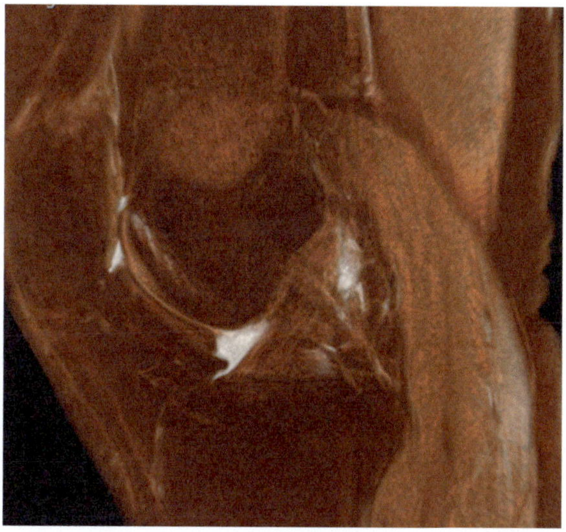

**Fig. 1** 3D MRI may facilitate the assessment of meniscal root and ACL integrity

coverage) may be present. MRI is also used to identify risk factors of ACLR failure including increased tibial slope [22], increased tibial cartilage slope, reduced middle cartilage area length, reduced MBA, femoral condyle geometry and narrow notch width. 3D MRI has been shown to increase the detection rate of ACL abnormalities and concomitant injuries including meniscal root injuries (Fig. 1).

Even though radiographs are not suitable for direct diagnosis of ACL injury, indirect signs based on bone abnormalities are of interest. Especially in the paediatric population, low velocity non-contact trauma is associated with ACL avulsion fractures. Early detection and ORIF are typically associated with satisfactory outcomes. The presence of a Segond´s fracture is thought to be pathognomonic for ACL injury. An arcuate fracture is associated with ACL injury. Osteochondral femoral impaction fractures are common but are associated with poor specificity and sensitivity. The extent of tibio-femoral subluxation and tibial slope can be assessed. As increased tibial slope has been shown to be associated with increased ACLR failure risk [39, 54, 59, 66, 85, 101, 153, 155, 194], radiographs are frequently used to assess tibial slope for the indication of slope correcting osteotomies. In addition to tibial slope, tunnel placement and biological processes in the setting of ACL revision surgery are typically assessed on radiographs. Computer tomography is typically used to assess 3-dimensional tunnel position for ACL revision planning.

# 3 Timing of ACLR

The timing of ACL reconstruction has clinical and socio-economic impact [133, 150]. The theoretical ideal moment for ACLR is when a graft is implanted into an optimal biological environment, where all concomitant injuries have resolved, and no consequential biological or mechanical alterations have occurred so that knee function can be restored ad integrum. Clinically applied, early ACLR will avoid unnecessary delay for return to full activity but has been shown to be associated with increased risk of arthrofibrosis. Delayed ACLR will minimise the risk of arthrofibrosis [150] and eventually emerge the necessity of the procedure but may be associated with consecutive chondral and/or meniscus tear and degeneration [69]. In addition, an emerging body of research is indicating that the tibial cartilage of the lateral compartment undergoes geometrical changes shortly after ACL injury which may increase the significance of supportive structures for rotatory knee stability. The individual assessment of the patient as well as the preoperative condition of the knee is important for correct timing of ACL reconstruction. ACL reconstruction is typically postponed several weeks until the acute intra-articular inflammatory phase is descendent, defined as the state where patients display under 5 degrees of extension deficit and at least 90 degrees of flexion with only moderate effusion and pain. ACL reconstruction should not be postponed more than 6 months in order to minimise the potential risk of consecutive chondral and or meniscal damage. In reality, elite athletes tend to undergo acute ACL reconstruction directly after ACL injury while just under 35% of ACL reconstructions in the amateur population are performed within 6 months following ACL injury. A growing body of research is indicating that acute ACL reconstruction in the setting of bucket-handle meniscus injuries is associated with satisfactory outcomes.

## 3.1 *Graft Choice and Clinical Implications*

As no specific graft has emerged to be exclusively superior to other grafts, graft choice is based on specific patient characteristics and expectations [8, 132, 139, 141, 162]. Graft choice defines kinetics and kinematics, biological response, donor site morbidity, knee function, stability, muscle balance, flexion/extension strength and recovery, RTS, overall patient satisfaction, risk-profile, complication rate, OA development, infection rate, psychological readiness, financial cost, operation time, as well as graft failure rate. While differences regarding some of the aforementioned parameters are not detected or eventually levelled out in the course of rehabilitation, other parameters including graft failure rate have been shown to be significantly different between grafts. A variety of grafts are available [140] including allografts, autografts and synthetic grafts. Most frequently used autografts comprise hamstring grafts, bone-patellar-tendon-bone grafts (BPTB), quadriceps tendon grafts (with or without bone block) as well as iliotibial band grafts. The most frequently used allografts include BPTB grafts, tibialis anterior/posterior tendon grafts, hamstring tendon grafts, achilles tendon grafts, iliotibial band grafts as well as peroneal tendon grafts. The role of allograft-ACL with retained anchor architecture remains unknown. Based on a current global benchmark study, the preferred grafts for primary ACL reconstruction are hamstring tendon autografts with 80.3%, BPTB autografts with 16.1%, quadriceps tendon autografts with 2.4% and allografts with 1% (Tuca 2023). Advantages of the latter in comparison to autografts include shorter surgical time, consistent implantation of robust grafts with predictable size, accelerated patient recovery and psychological readiness without donor site morbidity or harvesting-related complications. Typical concerns associated with the use of allografts include graft cost, risk of disease transmission, tissue weakening based on processing techniques, delayed graft incorporation based on immunologic responses, increased graft failure rates in the young active population and lower RTS rates compared to autografts. Hamstring, BPTB and QT autografts show typically no significant difference regarding overall patient satisfaction. However, relevant differences are of interest. Hamstring grafts have been shown to be associated with significantly increased graft failure rates when compared to BPTB grafts in the younger population. Even though hamstring grafts typically display superior tensile strength compared to BPTB and QT, they display lower young's modulus in the linear stress–strain curve area, especially in the young population [1]. As a result, the graft-bone interface is less stable during everyday knee kinematics with implications for biological processes and mechanical properties. The term hamstring graft is commonly used for grafts composed of the semitendinosus tendon and/or gracilis tendon even though the gracilis tendon is anatomically part of the adductor group. The unipennate gracilis muscle arises from the os pubis, while the partially uni and bipennate semitendinosus muscle arises from the tuber ischiadicum, which has implications for the direction of the tendon stripper during tendon harvest. The adductor group is innervated by the obturator nerve while the hamstring group being the *biceps femoris*, *semimembranosus* and *semitendinosus* is innervated by the sciatic nerve, which has implications for pain management following tendon harvest. Hamstring grafts are widely utilised because of their convenient characteristics [51] and strong tensile resistance which typically exceeds the tensile strength of the native ACL and all other most commonly used autografts. Hamstring tendons are easy to harvest and ensure easy graft passage without graft-tunnel length mismatch, show high tensile resistance, are compatible with all femoral fixation devices, show tolerable donor site morbidity and are associated with only few complications, the most common being saphenous nerve injury and premature graft amputation. In addition, hamstring tendons have the ability to regenerate, even though the quality of the regenerated tissue remains unknown. The downside of hamstring tendons are their unpredictable dimensions and maturity (even after preoperative MR assessment), as well as their significantly lower young's modulus, especially in younger patients. The elasticity or elasticity mismatch between semitendinosus and gracilis may affect biomechanical graft performance and biological graft incorporation. Time consuming graft preparation may be necessary in order to obtain a suitable graft and the cylindrical form of hamstring grafts increases the risk of PCL-impingement, consecutive activation of the reflex-arc, muscle inhibition and graft failure. Even though the diameter of a hamstring graft is highly correlated to ultimate tensile strength and young's modulus [56], there is conflicting evidence in the literature regarding the effect of hamstring graft size on risk of ACL revision surgery [40, 92, 96, 107]. Nevertheless, it is currently believed that the ideal hamstring graft should exceed 7.5 mm in diameter without producing any kind of impingement. As a 6 mm 4-stranded hamstring graft displays higher maximum load to failure compared to a 10 mm BTB graft [144], the graft diameter may not necessarily be the primary underlying reason for increased graft failure. Recently, the created tunnel area and direct fibre coverage are thought to play an important role in the longevity of a graft construct [114, 187]. The tunnel area created by a 10 mm reamer is twice the size compared to a 7 mm reamer. A tunnel with a diameter of 7 mm, located centrally in the femoral insertion area, may be associated with direct fibre coverage as low as 2.5 mm2. It has been hypothesised that femoral tunnel placement in the AM tunnel position may increase direct fibre coverage and eliminate the differences in ACLR failure rates based on graft diameter. However, decreased Young's modulus of hamstring grafts in the younger population is thought to affect the stability of the bone-tendon interface in biological healing processes. Based on several factors, increased failure rates associated with hamstring grafts compared to BPTB grafts in the younger population have been reported. If a tibial suspension system is used, a hamstring graft length of minimum 5.5 mm is thought to be necessary for graft incorporation. If a tibial interference screw is used, a longer graft is preferable as the fixation strength of the interference screw increases towards the external tunnel outlet where tibial bone density is highest. As folded grafts contain dead space, most grafts can be downsized by means of compression. A continuous loop device increases the top-diameter of the graft construct without affecting the graft mid-portion. As a result, the sizing of hamstring grafts may be associated with inaccuracy. A doubled semitendinosus/gracilis 4-strand-graft-construct typically displays a diameter between 7.7 and 8.5 mm [51]. Magnussen et al. found that grafts in the upper dimension with a diameter of 8.5 mm or more were associated with significantly decreased risk of ACL revision [92]. As a result, tripling or quadrupling of tendons is recommended and every further strand that is added to the graft construct increases the diameter of the final construct by approximately 0.75–1 mm. Depending on tendon length, there are numerous options for graft preparation [17, 41]. A tendon can be tripled by suturing the end of the tendon to a continuous loop device, pulling the free end through the loop and docking it into the created graft dale. The graft strands are equally tensioned and sutured to each other. With tripled grafts, a pulley-system can be used in order to ensure equal graft tension of the graft arms. The arms of a folded hamstring tendon show different resistance patterns and thus, different elongation percentage when tensioned with the same force. A significant mismatch may weaken the graft construct. The bone tendon interface healing is achieved through Sharpei fibres and aperture healing is thought to be a key feature of graft incorporation. Hamstring tendons change orientation within the tunnel through range of motion. While the direct fibres of the native ACL are bent through range of motion, hamstring tendon grafts with suspensory fixation rotate within the tunnel to a variable extent which may affect graft healing processes and incorporation. In terms of biological graft incorporation, BTPB grafts are superior to hamstring tendon grafts with biological healing phases of approximately 6 and 12 weeks, respectively. The prolonged biological graft incorporation phase of hamstring grafts is associated with increased anterior tibial translation in the early phase of rehabilitation compared to BPTB and QT. The knee adduction moment has been shown to be comparable following hamstring and BPTB graft harvest [181]. It is generally accepted that BPTB grafts represent the gold standard for ACL reconstruction in the young active patient with closed physes. Quadriceps tendon grafts are increasingly popular based on promising results in the younger population, displaying higher tensile strength and young's modulus compared to BPTB grafts and comparable donor site morbidity to hamstring grafts. In pure quadriceps tendon autografts, quadriceps tendon rupture must be considered as a rare complication. BPTB grafts have been found to be associated with increased donor site morbidity and risk of OA when compared to hamstring grafts. Bone-grafting the patellar defect from larger tibial bone blocks and minimal invasive techniques [148] are thought to eventually reduce donor site morbidity. In terms of complications, BPTB and quadriceps grafts display a more pronounced risk-profile compared to hamstring grafts. Complications associated with BPTB comprise patellar fracture, tibial fracture, patellar tendon rupture, patellar tendonitis and anterior knee pain. Complications associated with B-QT/QT comprise patella fracture or quadriceps tendon rupture. Complications associated with hamstring grafts are less common and detrimental, the most significant being saphenous nerve injury. In terms of infection rate, hamstring grafts have been associated with higher rates of infection compared to BPTB and QT based on increased risk of skin contact during graft harvest [2]. In terms of muscle function, BPTB and QT grafts weaken the extensor mechanism and are associated with temporary quadriceps muscle weakness. Hamstring grafts weaken the hamstring and/or adductor group which is associated with decreased flexion and adduction strength. The flexion strength deficit is typically present to some degree one year postoperatively but tends to resolve completely 5–6 years following ACL reconstruction in most cases. Hamstring grafts can be used in the skeletally immature patient in contrast to BPTB, where bone-block ingrowth into the physis may induce growth arrest. In terms of graft fixation, there is no consensus on knee angle or optimal graft tension. While excessive tension is thought to be associated with increased risk of ACL failure low tension may not sufficiently restore knee stability. The exact role of initial graft tension for final graft tension remains unknown. Most authors recommend between 20 and 90N initial graft tension. The initial tension pattern of a graft construct is dependent on several factors including graft preparation and fixation technique, applied graft tension, Young's modulus, graft orientation and knee flexion angle under graft fixation. The maximal sustained one-handed pull technique is currently the most used tensioning protocol [122]. However, the absolute tension applied varies from surgeon to surgeon [122]. In addition, significant loss of ACL graft force with tibial sided soft tissue interference screws has been observed 24 h following ACL implantation [78]. Myofibroblasts are thought to contribute to in-situ graft tension in the process of graft repopulation. The effect of graft pretensioning and initial graft tension on final graft properties remains unknown.

# 4 Graft Harvest

## *4.1 Hamstring Graft*

The gracilis tendon and semitendinosus tendon are identified at their junction at the pes anserinus. The knee is positioned in minimum 90 degrees of flexion. An oblique incision is made directly over the pes anserinus, and the sartorial fascia is exposed. A vertical incision increases the risk of damage to the infrapatellar branch of the saphenous nerve. The tendons can be palpated under the sartorius fascia. As the fascia is lifted with forceps, a vacuum is created, and a transversal roof is created which can be penetrated bluntly with Metzenbaum scissors. The Metzenbaum scissors are slid into the opening which is extended. Care must be taken not to damage parts of the saphenous nerve. The gracilis tendon and semitendinosus tendon can be visualised on the inside, adjacent to the lifted sartorius fascia. They can now be mobilised with a right angle. A cautious but tight pull will mobilise the tendons from adjacent tissue. A Langenbeck is introduced to visualise the tendons. Vinculae need to be transected to prevent tendon amputation. Each tendon is identified according to the anatomical position. The gracilis tendon is located cranially to the semitendinosus. A tendon stripper is mounted on the tendon to be released. If a substantial resistance is felt while advancing the stripper, the stripper should be removed, and the tendon should be inspected arthroscopically for vinculae which need to be detached. If the gastrocnemius muscle does not move while pulling the tendon, vinculae are typically sufficiently detached. Local anaesthetics can be given through a cannulated tendon stripper if available. Once the tendons are harvested, they can be inspected for utility. A gaze should be positioned between tendons and skin to minimise potential contamination. Muscle-tissue and unstable parts of the graft are removed. Recent studies have focussed on the effect of retaining muscle tissue, but results are inconclusive. The tendons are measured, and graft preparation is planned. To equalise tendon arms, tendon orientation is reversed with the proximal part of one tendon being adjacent to the distal part of the other. The ends of both grafts are whipstitched and prepared according to the corresponding fixation method.

## *4.2 Patella Tendon Graft*

With the knee in 90 degrees of flexion, a 5–8 cm longitudinal incision is made between the inferior border of the patella and the tibial tuberosity. The incision should be long enough to visualise both borders of the patellar tendon and to sufficiently mobilise the skin to access bone block areas. Placing the incision slightly medially to the midline may facilitate tibial bone drilling and eventually minimise pain when kneeling. The peritendineum is exposed through blunt dissection and incised longitudinally, hereby exposing the underlying patellar tendon. The mid-portion of the tendon is identified, and 2 longitudinal incisions are made from the patella down to the tibia, creating a 10 mm tendon strip. Bone block dimensions are marked with a marking pen. An oscillating saw with a small blade is used to cut the bone blocks. For the patella, a depth of 8–10 mm and a length of 20 mm is recommended. For the tibial bone block, a deeper cut can be made in order to harvest excessive bone which can be used to bone-graft the patella. The tip of the saw is typically angled towards the bone block in order to create a trapezoid bone block. The transversal cut can be divided into two cuts, creating a roof to minimise stress rising. When performing a single cut, the saw should be angled towards the bone block. The use of a mallet must be avoided in order to avoid patella fracture. Finally, the graft is sharply released from soft-tissue adherence and removed. Excessive bone is used to graft the patellar defect. For closure, the patellar tendon defect can be closed with single-knot sutures with the knee in flexion. The peritendineum should be closed with an absorbable running suture. Bone blocks are fashioned to fit to the corresponding bone tunnel dimension. Bone is typically removed and/or compressed. It is recommended to prepare and ensure easy graft passage. Excessive bone should be placed directly into the patellar defect, if possible, rather than be saved for the end of the operation. Two drill holes are made preferably in the cancellous bone portion of each bone block. Strong passing sutures are mounted on both bone blocks. It is advisable to mark the bone-tendon interface with a marking pen in order to confirm complete bone block entrance into the femoral tunnel. A potential tunnel-graft mismatch should be avoided. A suitable instrument is used to facilitate bone block exit out of the tibial tunnel and entrance into the femoral tunnel. The graft is then typically secured with an interference screw or by suspensory fixation methods. Screw divergence should be avoided based on potential graft damage, bone-block amputation as well as reduced fixation strength. The use of reverse threaded screws may avoid the graft to rotate anteriorly in right knees and has been shown to be associated with reduced laxity compared to normally threaded screws at 12 months follow up [112].

## *4.3 Quadriceps Tendon Graft*

The dimension and location of the incision for quadriceps tendon harvest is dependent on the harvesting technique with corresponding instruments. The following technique describes the use of mini-invasive instruments. With the knee in 90 degrees of flexion, a 3–5 cm longitudinal incision is made from the proximal border of the patella, extending proximally following the quadriceps muscle course. The peritendineum is visualised through blunt dissection. A gaze can be used to gently release subcutaneous fat tissue. The peritendineum is incised, exposing the underlying quadriceps tendon. The portion of the tendon which lies in line with the mid-portion of the patella is identified. A U-shaped quadriceps-harvesting knife is inserted into the mid-portion of the tendon in close proximity to the patella and advanced minimum 7 cm proximally in line with the tendon. Care must be taken to follow the natural course of the tendon fibres and avoid muscle damage. The created cut is inspected for completeness and re-cut if necessary. The arthroscope can be advanced into the opening for visualisation.

The vertical border of the tendon strip close to the patella is visualised and a second harvesting knife with a transverse caudal blade is inserted perpendicularly into the vertical tendon portion. The transversal caudal blade is inserted to create a 5 mm thick tendon graft, penetrating the opposite tendon border at equal depth. The tendon knife is then advanced in the same manner as the first. Complete caudal-longitudinal release of the tendon is verified. A third release knife is inserted and advanced to the proximal end of the tendon strip. Care must be taken not to activate the release knife while advancing it. The tendon strip is released proximally and removed. A gaze is placed around the tendon to avoid contamination through skin contact. If a bone block is planned, the bone block dimensions are marked with a marking pen. An oscillating saw with a small blade is used to cut the bone block with a depth of 8–10 mm and a length of approximately 20 mm. The tip of the saw is angled towards the bone block in order to create a trapezoid bone block. The transversal cut can be divided into two cuts, creating a roof to minimise stress rising. When performing a single cut, the tip of the saw should be angled towards the bone block. The use of a mallet must be avoided in order to avoid patella fracture. If the bone block cannot be easily mobilised with an osteotome, it is advisable to re-cut the bone block with emphasis on the corners. However, cross cutting should be avoided as it has been found to be associated with increased risk of patella fracture under rehabilitation. Finally, the graft is sharply released from soft-tissue and removed. Excessive bone is used to bone-graft the patellar defect. The peritendineum can be closed with an absorbable running suture. The bone block is fashioned to fit to the corresponding bone tunnel dimension. Bone is typically removed and/or compressed. It is recommended to prepare and ensure easy graft passage. Excessive bone should be placed directly into the patellar defect, if possible, rather than be saved for the end of the operation. Two drill holes are made preferably parallel to the cortex in the cancellous portion of the bone block. Strong passing sutures are mounted on the bone block. The tendon portion is whipstitched with high-tensile suture material. It is advisable to mark the bone-tendon junction with a marking pen in order to confirm correct graft position and orientation. The graft is then ready for implantation. A suitable instrument can be used to facilitate bone block exit out of the tibial tunnel and entrance into the femoral tunnel. The graft is then typically secured with an interference screw or by suspensory fixation methods. Screw divergence should be avoided based on potential graft damage, bone-block amputation as well as reduced fixation strength. The use of reverse threaded screws may avoid the graft to rotate anteriorly in right knees and has been shown to be associated with reduced laxity compared to normally threaded screws at 12 months follow up [112].

## 5 Femoral Tunnel Placement

Femoral tunnel placement has received substantial scientific attention in recent years [68, 71, 99, 109, 147, 185, 183] as femoral tunnel malpositioning is thought to be the most common cause of technical ACLR failure and subsequent ACL revision surgery.

The difficulty associated with precise femoral tunnel placement is based on inconsistent or indistinct landmarks, arthroscopic image distortion [64, 65], 2-dimensional monitor visualisation of a 3 dimensional complex, anatomic variability and significant changes in anatomic appearance based on knee flexion angle. In addition to difficulties with tunnel precision (consistent tunnel location), tunnel accuracy (correct tunnel location) is still a matter of scientific debate. There is a broad consensus among knee surgeons on anatomic tunnel positioning, i.e. tunnel positioning within the native ACL insertion area. As approximately only two-thirds of the femoral insertion area is covered with standard tunnel reaming, native ACL insertions are currently not reproduced with single bundle ACL reconstruction techniques. Even a 10 mm reamer with a 50-degree drill angle will produce a tunnel of less diameter than most femoral insertion areas. As a result, double bundle ACLR has been recommended for femoral insertional sites exceeding 14 mm using a 5.5 mm HT graft for the AM position and a 5 mm HT graft for the PL bundle. Several studies have failed to show clear superiority of DB ACLR compared to single bundle ACL reconstruction. Different positions within the ACL insertion area have different properties. Factors that need to be considered comprise graft longevity [102] and biological processes, overall performance and stabilising properties. Currently, the central femoral footprint position and the eccentric high AM position are the most commonly used positions for femoral tunnel placement. The central femoral footprint position aims at the overall ACL femoral insertion site which is thought to be located 6.1 mm posterior to the lateral intercondylar ridge, 14.7 mm proximal to the distal cartilage margin and 8.5 mm anterior to the posterior cartilage margin. The mean distance from the lateral intercondylar ridge to the inferior articular cartilage margin has been shown to be 10.1 mm [12]. The attributes of the eccentric AM bundle position are summarised in the apronym I.D.E.A.L., i.e. **i**sometric, located in the area of **d**irect fibres, **e**ccentrically but within the **a**natomic footprint, thus exposed to **l**ow tension. An increasing body of research is emphasising that increased ACL direct insertion coverage is associated with positive biomechanical effects [186, 187]. The percent of direct fibre coverage is dependent on tunnel centre, drill diameter and drill angle. As the tunnel area increases non-linearly based on the diameter of the reamer, a tunnel of 10 mm diameter has approximately twice the aperture size of a tunnel of 7 mm diameter. It has been hypothesised that even though hamstring grafts show higher tensile strength compared to most other autografts, the tendency towards smaller tunnel diameters and eccentric low functional graft position within the tunnel result in less coverage of the direct fibre insertion. The direct insertion with its 4 layered anchor architecture is located adjacent to the lateral intercondylar ridge (resident's ridge) and has been found to show significant variation in size and proportion but is most frequently described to be approximately 5 mm in width. The four layers being bone, mineralised fibrocartilage, non-mineralised fibrocartilage and ligament gradually transduce force between the elastic ligament and the rigid bone. The four layered anchor architecture is typically not restored by current ACLR techniques. The femoral ACL insertion observed macroscopically corresponds typically to the direct insertion observed microscopically. In several cases, the direct insertion has been shown to be relatively narrow and small diameter reamers with posterior (low) positioning may completely avoid the direct insertion. The indirect insertion which is adjacent to the inferior articular cartilage margin appears membrane-like and is composed of fibres which are attached to the bone in a more parallel manner through a less aggressive 2-layer anchor architecture. The biomechanical effectiveness of grafts positioned perpendicularly in the area of the indirect insertion area is currently elucidated but remains unclear. In order to maximise coverage of the direct insertion, the tunnel centre should be positioned close to the lateral intercondylar ridge. The proportion of direct and indirect insertion has been shown to be highly variable and thus, without assessment of the contralateral knee or the presence of a distinct femoral remnant, the exact dimension of the direct insertion area remains unknown. For orientation in the proximal–distal dimension, the bifurcate ridge represents an important bony landmark, separating the AM from the PL bundle, albeit only identifiable in approximately 50% of the cases. Grafts placed at the AM bundle position near the femoral back wall junction undergo minimal lengthening through ROM, tensioning insignificantly in flexion. Grafts placed at the PL bundle position show significant tightening in extension. It has been hypothesised that (near)- isometric graft behaviour may facilitate biological graft healing, which is thought to be one reason for increased graft longevity found for grafts placed at the AM bundle position compared to the central footprint position [23, 193]. Arthroscopically, femoral tunnel placement is typically based on bony and soft tissue landmarks. Bony landmarks for femoral tunnel placement comprise the lateral intercondylar ridge (resident's ridge), the bifurcate ridge, the femoral notch roof, the over-the-top position and the posterior notch outlet. Other important landmarks are the posterior horn of the lateral meniscus [71] and the posterior cartilage-bone junction. The lateral intercondylar ridge (resident's ridge) has been found to be a reliable bony landmark after non-mechanical removal of soft tissue and can also be identified through fluoroscopy. The lateral intercondylar ridge is of particular interest as it represents the anterior border of the ACL insertion area, facilitating orientation in the anterior–posterior dimension. The course of the posterior femoral bony margin has the form of a slide with variable slope. This specific condylar geometry associates proximal tunnel placement with anterior tunnel placement (going up the slide) and posterior tunnel placement with distal tunnel placement (going down the slide). As a result, moderately proximally placed tunnels tend to display more AM direct fibre coverage than tunnels placed centrally in the femoral insertion area. The posterior cartilage-bone junction has been found to be a reliable landmark in conjunction with tangents defining notch dimension: a line connecting the most distal high shallow point with the most proximal high deep point of the notch defines the length of the notch. A perpendicular line connects the junction-line with the lowest point of the cartilage-margin and defines the height of the notch (Fig. 2).

The femoral insertion is found close to the intersection of to tangents: a tangent from the over-the-top-position to the lowest point of the cartilage margin; and a tangent from the posterior cartilage bone junction to the most distal high shallow point of the notch. The s-shaped contour of the posterior condyle shows variations, especially in regard to the distance of the cartilage-bone junction to the condylar wall-roof junction. The posterior horn of the lateral meniscus in hyper-flexion has been

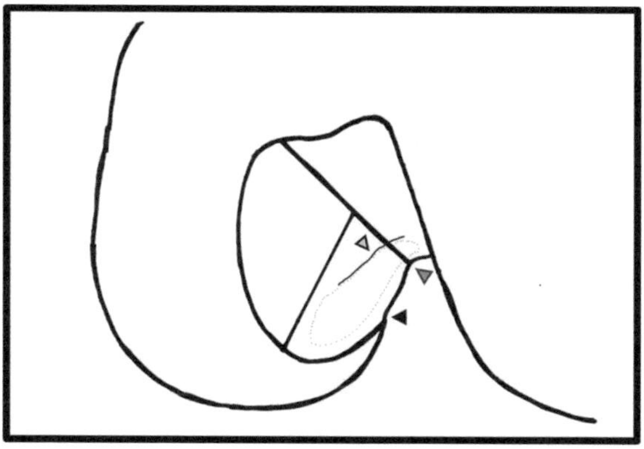

**Fig. 2** A schematic arthroscopic view of the medial aspect of the lateral femoral condyle. The blue arrow marks the condylar wall-roof junction. A line connecting the most distal high shallow point with the most proximal high deep point of the notch defines the length of the notch. A perpendicular line connects the junction-line with the lowest point of the cartilage-margin and defines the height of the notch wall (adapted from [90]). The green arrow marks a schematic view of the resident's ridge. The black arrow marks the cartilage-bone junction

shown to be a reliable landmark for femoral tunnel placement [183]. The centre of the femoral tunnel does not correspond to the functional graft position and associated biomechanical properties [3]. When bone blocks are used, an interference screw will typically compress the bone block to a relatively narrow area diametral opposed to the position of the screw. Therefore, the tunnel centre must be adapted to the intended functional graft position. If the functional graft position is intended to be within the direct insertion area and an interference screw is planned to be positioned *above* the graft, the tunnel centre must be located anterior to the ACL insertion. Conversely, if a hamstring graft is used with suspensory fixation, the tunnel centre must be located within the direct insertion area. This concept is further complicated by the fact that hamstring grafts have been shown to display eccentric positions within the tunnel with further changes of position through range of motion. Femoral tunnel placement can be assessed radiologically and objectified by the quadrant method [10, 68, 105]. The Blumensaat's line can be divided into four equal quadrants. The femoral tunnel should be located in the most posterior quadrant. On a superposed rectangular grid, the centre of the ACL insertion area is thought to be located 34% posterior to the Blumensaat's line and 27% anterior to the posterior border of the femoral cortex on the grid. Recently, the use of compressed MRI-sequences resembling a lateral x-ray image have gained attention to identify the femoral insertion area preoperatively. The femoral insertion area can then be re-identified intraoperatively through fluoroscopy. Based on a distorted, two-dimensional view of the knee in standard arthroscopy, typical landmarks and descriptions of ACL native insertion areas do not ensure anatomical orientation and consecutive precise tunnel placement. As a result, non-anatomic femoral tunnel placement is thought to represent the main cause of technical error as observed in ACL revision surgery. In the future, technology assisted tunnel placement may increase the precision of tunnel placement through quantitative geometric data of ACL attachments. In addition, anatomic techniques are required to accurately reproduce the native ACL insertion area including fibre-restoration extending from the cartilage margin into the notch roof.

## 6 Tibial Tunnel Placement

Tibial tunnel placement has received less scientific attention compared to femoral tunnel placement, even though the morphology of the tibial ACL insertion area has been thoroughly revisited. The appearance of the tibial ACL insertion is associated to significant variability but typically described as an oval, triangular or c-shaped formation, bounded posteriorly by the medial and lateral intercondylar tubercles, anteriorly by the Parson's knob, medially by the medial intercondylar ridge and laterally by the anterior horn of the lateral meniscus. The tibial insertion site is thought to comprise two bundle areas. The crescent shaped AM insertion area is located along an L-shaped formation constituted by the Parson's knob and the medial intercondylar ridge, enfolding the smaller PL insertion area which is located diametrically close to the lateral tibial spine. The resulting bundle division has a posteromedial-to-anterolateral course. The centre of the tibial insertion site is thought to be located 10.5 mm posterior to the Parson's knob, 13 mm anterior to the retro-eminence ridge and 7.5 mm medial to the anterior horn of the lateral meniscus. The anterior aspect of the anterior horn of the lateral meniscus is in line with the AM bundle insertion. The fibrous attachments of the posterior aspect of the anterior horn of the lateral meniscus are in line with the PL bundle insertion. The anterior intermeniscal ligament is located 9.1 mm anterior from the centre of the tibial insertion area. The ACL insertion is located 7 mm anterior to the PCL. Recent anatomical studies with emphasis on meticulous removal of synovial coverage and connective tissue have failed to identify a functional posterolateral portion of the ACL and describe the tibial insertion area as a continuous c-shaped, double-c-shaped or J-shaped anteromedial insertion. Direct fibres form a curved narrow anteromedial insertion along the medial intercondylar ridge and the Parson's Knob while indirect fibres extend anteriorly to complete the 3-dimensional duck-foot appearance of the tibial ACL insertion site. Both the anterior and posterior horn of the lateral meniscus blend into the c-shaped tibial ACL insertion area, which has been hypothesised to have implications for ACL kinetics based on meniscal movement and position. Even though the anatomy of the tibial plateau is well described, arthroscopic landmarks such as the posterior edge of the anterior horn of the lateral meniscus and even the use of the ACL remnant have failed to reproduce tibial tunnels with a consistent percentage of the antero-posterior tibial diameter. During ACLR, in most cases an ACL remnant can be identified. The remnant has typically retained synovial coverage but changed orientation and undergone morphological changes. Based on the convergence of the guide-pin and the course of the native ACL, a guide pin that penetrates the centre of the ACL remnant creates a tunnel which lies posterior to the insertional centre of the remnant. Similarly, the posterior edge of the anterior horn of the lateral meniscus as a landmark for tibia tunnel placement is not reliable. In cases in which the lateral compartment is subluxed, meniscal position may be altered. As a result, lateral femoro-tibial displacement has been shown to be associated with more posterior tibial tunnel placement. Radiologically, the position of tibial ACL bundle insertion areas and tibial tunnels are expressed as the percentage of the anterior–posterior (AP) tibial diameter. However, the correct radiological position of ACL bundles is still a matter of scientific debate. For the most part, the AM bundle is thought to be located at 36% of the tibial AP diameter while the PL bundle is thought to be located at 52% of the tibial AP tibial diameter. The optimal tibial tunnel position for single bundle ACL reconstruction also varies in the literature ranging from 35 to 48% of the AP tibial diameter. The broadest consensus on tibial tunnel placement has been that the centre of the tibial tunnel should be located at 40% of the medial-to-lateral width of the interspinous distance, in line with the posterior edge of the lateral meniscus anterior horn, approximately 15 mm anterior to the posterior cruciate ligament. However, an increasing body of evidence is emphasising that more anteriorly placed grafts are associated with superior biomechanical properties. The trend is reflected by the fact that high volume ACL surgeons tend to place tibial tunnels more anteriorly compared to low volume surgeons. A novel approach comprises preoperative individual MRI assessment of tibial landmarks and their unique geometry and constellation in order to reliably reproduce tibial tunnel placement. Especially the spatial proximity of the posterior edge of the anterior horn of the lateral meniscus to the centre of the ACL remnant should be assessed preoperatively. The ACL insertion area shows significant variability and individual assessment of the specific insertional anatomy is gaining scientific attention. Fluoroscopy facilitates consistent tunnel placement in terms of as a percentage of the AP tibial diameter but does not account for individual insertional morphology. A preoperative construct displaying individual insertional morphology is needed for optimal tunnel placement. Recently, it has been shown possible to compress MRI sequences into a single image, resembling a lateral x-ray, in order to identify the exact location of the tibial insertion area. The area can then be re-identified under fluoroscopy [167]. The centre of the tibial tunnel does not correspond to the functional graft position within the tunnel. In addition, the position of the interference screw within the tibial tunnel has shown to affect the obliquity of the graft. A posterolateral screw position is advisable in order to position the graft in an anteromedial position. When creating the tibial tunnel, sequential drilling is thought to increase the precision of the tunnel position. If the guide-wire is slightly off the intended position, the guide pin can be over-drilled with 4.5 mm drill and adjusted to an optimised position. The guide pin is hereafter drilled into the femoral roof and over-drilled with the intended drill diameter. Holding the guide wire with a clamp while drilling is not advisable as metal particles are typically released into joints which can induce inflammatory processes. Tibial fixation is thought to be the weakest link of a graft construct based on the lower bone mineral density of the proximal tibia compared with the distal femur and the force vector of applying forces on the graft.

## 7 ACL Graft Healing

The mechanisms of ACL graft healing are not yet fully understood. Current knowledge is derived from animal studies, MRI assessment and in vivo biopsy studies which are associated with variable findings [189, 191]. Essential processes of hamstring tendon graft healing include bone-tendon healing and mid-substance graft remodelling [176]. Tendon-bone interfaces as well as the graft mid-substance are exposed to different biological environments and biomechanical impact, undergoing different but coordinated healing mechanisms. Concurrent and consecutive biological processes define the weakest link of the graft construct which is progressively shifted from the bone-tendon interface towards the mid-substance of the graft. Central and unsolved challenge regarding bone-tendon healing is the restoration of the 4-layered direct ACL anchor architecture. Central challenge of mid-substance remodelling is the formation and maintenance of adequate graft-tension through the process of gradual cell necrosis and graft repopulation through myofibroblasts. After graft implantation, an immediate inflammatory response is triggered and neutrophils and macrophages from the synovial fluid are recruited to the periphery of the graft construct. The graft undergoes gradual cell necrosis and disintegration of collagen fibrils which induces gradually increasing laxity of the graft construct, but also the release of growth factors which stimulate cell migration. Increased levels of interleukin-6, TNF-alpha, transforming growth factor-beta as well as matrix-metalloproteinase-1 levels are typically observed. The attracted mesenchymal stem cells repopulate the graft and produce endothelial growth factor (VEGF) to control re-vascularisation. The vasculature is thought to originate from the synovium, corpus Hoffa and infra-patellar plica. Fibroblasts which can endure the synovial fluid, synthesise extra-cellular graft products. Myofibroblasts are thought to define graft tension. Differentiated mesenchymal stem cells produce extracellular matrix and remodelling enzymes in order to establish a firm tendon-bone interface through Sharpey fibres at the bone-tendon interface. Even though completed osseo-integration of grafts with formation of multilayered tendon-to-bone interfaces has been observed, the majority of studies suggest the formation of a simple fibrous anchor architecture through Sharpey fibres with non-uniform healing. The process is preceded by the formation of a fibrovascular interface within the tunnels and is thought to coincide with the inflammation and proliferation phase of the graft mid-substance. Failure to establish a fibrovascular interface due to excessive inflammation and catalytic processes may result in graft pull out and is thought to be one of the primary causes of ACL graft failure at early stages of rehabilitation. For graft fixation with suspensory fixation, graft movement within the tunnel and the young's modulus of a given graft may play a role in the stability of the tendon-bone interface and formation of the fibrovascular interface. However, the formation of a stable tendon-bone interface is not strictly necessary for stability of a graft construct if fixation hardware is fully functional. Excellent short term clinical results without evidence of osseo-integration or connecting fibres at the femoral tendon–bone interface have been observed (Nebelung) [115]. The inflammatory response is thought to have a substantial impact on ACLR healing. In addition, clinical outcomes of ACLR have been shown to be associated with the nature of the inflammatory response of the knee following ACL injury as well as ACLR. Increased concentrations of IL-6 and MMP3 in the synovial fluid early after ACL injury have been shown to be associated with compromised gait biomechanics 6 months following ACLR [36]. Graft loosening has been shown to be associated with increased gene and protein expression of IL-6, IL-8 and TNF-alpha within the first year of ACLR. Bone tunnel enlargement has been shown to be associated with elevated synovial fluid concentrations of IL-1-beta [27]. Increased levels of IL-1-alpha concentrations on the day of surgery have been shown to be associated with lower IKDC scores [82]. The maturation of the fibrovascular interface to a definite anchor architecture is thought to represent an important step of ACL graft healing. However, the 4-layered force transducing direct anchor architecture of the native ACL is typically not regenerated. Instead, a non-uniform indirect anchor architecture through Sharpey fibres is typically observed. The fibrocartilage layers in the native direct insertion contain glycosaminoglycans (GAG) which are thought to provide tissue elasticity and resistance to tensile, shear and compressive forces. Unloading and immobilisation typically induces chondrocyte apoptosis, decreased chondrocyte proliferation and decreased GAG´s in fibrocartilage layers. The tidemark between the mineralized and unmineralized fibrocartilage of the direct insertion is of particular interest as it marks a mechanical boundary which is thought to reduce damage to soft tissues during joint movement. In addition, it marks a nutritious barrier. Mechanical stress is thought to be important for the development of fibrocartilage. Increased chondrocytes at the tendon-bone interface may be decisive for the formation of fibrocartilage layers. Appropriate mechanical stress of the tendon-bone interface is thought to be important for maturation. As long as the insertional microarchitecture of the ACL is not replaced or regenerated through ACLR techniques, altered biomechanics must be expected.

## 8 ACL Repair

In synergy with refined anatomical, biological and biomechanical understanding of the ACL, the concept of ACL repair has regained significant scientific attention in recent years [35, 38, 126, 136]. The renewed interest in ACL repair is based on advances in surgical techniques and the evidence of intrinsic ACL healing potential [13]. The exact healing process of the ACL is not yet fully understood but to some extent analogous to the intrinsic healing mechanism of the MCL undergoing a firm reattachment and displaying disorganised collagen fibres, neovascularization, myofibroblasts and collagen type III. The epiligament of the ACL merges with the periosteum at the ACL insertion sites and is thought to play an important role in the process of ACL healing by controlling water and metabolite influx and providing cells and vasculature [44]. ACL repair has historically always been of interest based on its less invasive nature compared to ACLR while retaining native ligament characteristics.

However, the challenge of stable and sufficient healing which translates to satisfactory re-rupture rates remains unsolved. Rigorous patient selection, systematic injury assessment, meticulous surgical technique and structured rehabilitation are thought to be key features of successful ACL repair. The current classification by Sherman is based on the extent of remaining tissue on the femur and comprises four types from minimal remaining tissue to mid-substance tears. Sherman type I tears represent true soft tissue avulsions with minimal tissue remaining on the femur. Sherman type II tears display approximately up to 20% remaining tissue. Sherman type III tears display approximately up to 33% remaining tissue on the femur and Sherman type IV tears are true mid-substance tears. ACL repair is commonly recommended for Sherman type I and II ACL injuries. A central aspect of ACL repair is the direct insertion of the native ACL. The 4-layered direct insertion comprises the following layers: bone, mineralised fibrocartilage, fibrocartilage and ligament. The stiffness gradient is thought to transduce forces progressively and allow for fibril recruitment. Between the mineralised fibrocartilage and fibrocartilage, a tidemark is typically seen. The tidemark is of particular interest as it marks a mechanical boundary which is thought to reduce damage to soft tissues during joint movement. In addition, it marks a nutritious barrier. While the mineralised fibrocartilage is vascularised by the bony side, the fibrocartilage is vascularised by the joint side. If vasculature is compromised, tissue from the rupture site to the tidemark may be compromised. Mechanical stress is thought to be important for the development of fibrocartilage. The fibrocartilage layers in the native direct insertion contains glycosaminoglycans (GAG) which are thought to provide tissue elasticity and resistance to tensile, shear and compressive forces (Sakane). Unloading and immobilisation typically induces chondrocyte apoptosis, decreased chondrocyte proliferation and decreased GAG´s in fibrocartilage layers. Based on current findings in animal studies, the presence of chondrocytes may be important for the restoration of the direct insertion. The fine balance between structural stability and appropriate mechanical stress following ACL repair is thought to be an important factor for ACL healing mechanisms. Other classifications have been established, e.g. the three-digit ACL rupture classification. The first digit describes the rupture location of the ACL being proximal (A), central (B) or distal (C). The second digit describes rupture morphology affecting 1 bundle (1), 2 bundles (2) or being multi-lacerated (3). The third digit describes the ACL synovial tube being completely intact (1), $\geq$ 50% intact (2) or $<$ 50% intact (3). The status of the synovial tube may indicate the status of the epiligament. The presence of type III collagen plays an important role in healing mechanisms and neovascularization. The proximity of the rupture to the insertional areas with collagen type III presence may play a decisive for role for healing potential. Also, the integrity and cellular density of the epiligament may be of paramount importance for healing potential. Arthroscopic ACL repair typically involves a self-retrieving looped suture which is passed through the distal ACL stump in order to re-attach the ACL stump to the femoral insertion area with a suture anchor or suspensory cortical fixation. Adjustable tensioning loops as well as suture tape augmentation have been shown to biomechanically support the construct, reducing the risk of cyclic displacement and failure. There are ongoing concerns of inflammatory responses and lack of data regarding eventual undesirable long-term effects. Dynamic intraligamentary stabilisation (DIS) DIS, in which a non-resorbable suture is fixed to a tibial spring implant, represents a viable alternative. The spring implant induces a posterior drawer-type force, protecting [156] the repaired ACL graft. However, even though comparable results of DIS and other techniques have been described in the literature, DIS is typically associated with increased risk of hardware complications and two staged revision in case of failure [136]. Even though the efficiency of biological augmentation on surgical outcomes of ACL repair is unclear, PRP, collagen-scaffolds and micro-fracture are thought to enhance the healing potential of the ACL. LEAP´s are currently considered to aid in the biological healing process by attuning joint kinematics [38].

## 9 ACL Augmentation

Partial ACL injuries are observed in 10–27% of isolated ACL injuries [24]. Based on uncharacteristic symptomatology and reduced imaging accuracy, partial ACL injuries represent a diagnostic challenge and are believed to be underreported. The percentage of partial ACL injuries progressing to complete ACL injuries as well as the percentage of partial ACL injuries becoming asymptomatic are unknown. ACL augmentation is indicated if the remaining bundle is functional [33, 170]. To date, no constellation of clinical tests is thought to reliably detect isolated bundle insufficiency and even arthroscopic evaluation, which is thought to be the gold standard for the diagnosis of partial ACL injury, does not reliably discriminate bundle, epiligament or anchor architecture integrity. Despite a sound theoretical foundation, ACL augmentation is thought to be reserved for special cases and conventional ACL reconstruction is recommended for nonfunctional partial ACL injuries or cases in which the functionality of the remaining bundle cannot be completely verified. ACL augmentation consists of reconstruction of the compromised bundle while preserving the functional bundle.

## 10 Double Bundle ACL Reconstruction

On a theoretical level, anatomic double bundle ACL reconstruction is commonly regarded to be superior to single bundle ACL reconstruction based on a more complete anatomic bundle restoration [19, 75]. However, tissue gradients, bundle interaction, fibre bending mechanisms, insertional microarchitecture and other factors associated with native biomechanics of the ACL are typically not addressed. There is conflicting evidence in the literature regarding superiority of double bundle ACL reconstruction in regard to subjective and objective outcomes in the unselected population compared to single bundle ACL reconstruction. A recent meta-analysis reported no difference in knee stability, clinical function, graft failure rate as well as OA changes with a follow up of minimum 5 years [21]. A meta-analysis by Oh et al. reported superiority of double bundle ACL reconstruction in regard to anteroposterior stability without affecting rotatory laxity [123]. While time zero biomechanical studies tend to favour double bundle ACL reconstruction over single bundle ACL reconstruction [136], long term functional outcomes tend to be similar between double bundle and single bundle ACL reconstruction. In addition, as double bundle ACL reconstruction is technically demanding and may represent a challenge in the setting of revision ACLR, double bundle ACL reconstruction in the unselected population is currently not recommended. Double bundle ACL reconstruction involves typically the use of the gracilis and semitendinosus tendon for the implantation of two distinct grafts. Small insertional areas are not suitable for double bundle ACL reconstruction. Tibial tunnels are established based on the anatomic ACL insertional area with an anteromedial and posterolateral tunnel. A guide pin is inserted into the centre of the AM bundle medial to the posterior margin of the anterior horn of the lateral meniscus, in close proximity to the Parson's knob. A second guide pin is inserted in the centre of the PL bundle just medial to the lateral tibial spine. The tunnel apertures should display an adequate distance to avoid tunnel merging. According to graft diameter and based on insertional morphology, adequately sized reamers are used to establish bone tunnels. Tibial tunnels can be merged distally through a 10 mm reamer creating a common tunnel stem, given the outer tibial entry points are planned accordingly [146]. The branched double bundle ACL reconstruction technique is thought to be associated with less injury to intra articular structures, less synovial fluid passage and less unwanted biological reactions. The femoral tunnels are typically created through the AM portal with a free hand technique or through a guided out-side-in technique. If arthroscopic landmarks are unclear, the AM tunnel is created as close as possible to the condylar back-wall on the medial wall of the lateral condyle. A line from the cartilage-bone junction to the most distal-high point of the notch typically bisects the tunnel aperture. The PL tunnel is created on a tangent from the over-the-top-position to the deepest point of the condylar cartilage margin. An adequate distance between tunnel apertures is needed to avoid tunnel merging and ensure sufficient mechanical graft fixation properties. Tendons are prepared accordingly and implanted. The fixation angle and tension for graft fixation is still a matter of scientific debate [131]. Increasing the PL bundle fixation angle has been shown to correlate with improvement of the pivot-shift phenomenon in cadaveric knees [131]. Fixation angles of the AM and PL bundle of 20 and 45 degrees of flexion, respectively, have been shown to be associated with improved function compared to single bundle reconstruction based on in vivo laboratory models [75]. Järvelä et al. reported improved rotational stability of patients undergoing double bundle ACL reconstruction with fixation angles of the AM and PL bundle of 30 and 0 degrees of flexion, respectively, when compared to single bundle ACL reconstruction at 2 years follow up [70]. However, the significant between-group difference in rotational stability was no longer observed at 5 years follow up. Further research is needed to ultimately determine the role and relevance of double-bundle ACL reconstruction in the future.

## 11 Rehabilitation After ACL Reconstruction

Rehabilitation following ACLR comprises a musculoskeletal, neurophysiological and psychological dimension [6]. Current rehabilitation programs emphasise an immediate structured progressive approach as several key mechanisms of successful ACLR including restoration of neuromuscular control as well as biological healing processes are thought to be dependent on appropriate mechanical stress. The pace of progression is typically dependent on several factors including level of function, type of sport, graft choice, concomitant injuries, profession, response to surgery, psychological status and pain perception. Rehabilitation following ACLR intends to restore ROM, enhance muscle strength, proprioception, functional stability and psychological readiness for RTS. The resulting target is the combination of the highest possible functional level and the lowest possible re-injury risk for the patient. Central aspects of the progressive sequence of rehabilitation can be summarised through the apronym WORLD-CUP. **W**alking, **O**ne-legged squatting, **R**unning, **L**anding, **D**ecelerating/dropping, **CU**tting, **P**laying. The goal of rehabilitation in the primary immediate phase after ACLR is the management of the inflammatory response of the knee to surgery. Main target is the normalisation of the gait cycle based on the reduction of swelling and pain, limitation of arthrogenic muscle inhibition as well as graft protection. Typical interventions are ice, compression, elevation and ROM exercises. Weight bearing is typically allowed in the absence of significant pain and effusion in accordance with relevant concomitant injury protocols. Braces may be used in specific cases, e.g. in the setting of concomitant meniscal root repair. Patella mobilisation is encouraged in the setting of BPTB-graft harvest. Terminal extension based on confident quadriceps recruitment and control in the absence of swelling and pain is fundamental for further progression. In secondary phases, the safe progression in the rehabilitation sequence by promotion of kinematic patterns with increasing loading, velocity and complexity are of interest. Primary target is a strong and controlled near-normalised simultaneous hip, knee and ankle flexion in combination with core stability. Two-legged squats are introduced to gain strength and to refine the technique. In the following, one-legged squats are introduced which are thought to be fundamental for further progression towards high velocity kinematics. In tertiary phases of the rehabilitation sequence, the resumption of running is prepared. The confidence to swing and load the knee unrestrictedly with sufficient strength and control is thought to represent a neurophysiological and psychological breakthrough. Plyometric training is introduced to maximise the development of speed and power. One legged landing is thought to be of kinematic importance as it not only represents the ability to absorb forces, but more importantly, a potential motion of injury. Optimising landing techniques is thought to be of paramount importance for the reduction of ACL re-injury risk. In the course of rehabilitation, one-legged drop jumps and cutting manoeuvres are introduced. A central aspect of rehabilitation is the controlled simulation of sports with progressive sport-specific movements and scenarios. The final aspect of rehabilitation involves the transition from a controlled training environment towards a non-foreseeable chaotic free-play environment. Detailed description of protocols and their effectiveness can be found in the literature.

## 12 Complications of ACL Reconstruction

Complications of ACLR comprise complications arising from preoperative factors, the surgery itself and the course of rehabilitation [169]. Complications arising from preoperative factors include surgical planning and timing. Early ACLR is believed to be associated with increased risk of arthrofibrosis. Even though there is conflicting evidence on the association of early ACLR and arthrofibrosis, excessive inflammatory responses following ACLR have been shown to negatively affect functional outcomes and induce loss of motion. Aggressive rehabilitation, manipulation under anaesthesia and/or lysis of adhesions may be indicated depending on the severity of the complication. The extensive release of severe posterior capsular adhesion has been shown to be associated with satisfactory outcomes. Delayed ACLR in the unstable knee has been shown to be associated with increased risk of irreparable meniscus and cartilage pathology. Meniscal transplantation and advanced cartilage surgery may be indicated in special cases. The diagnosis of ACL insufficiency is typically made through anamnesis, clinical examination and MRI. However, cases in which functional ACL´s are removed based on poor diagnosis have been reported. Neglected pathology is thought to represent one of the common complications of ACLR. Especially overlooked MCL, PLC and meniscal injuries may be associated with persisting pain, instability and increased risk of mechanical ACL graft failure. Complications arising from the surgery itself include complications associated with graft harvest, tunnel placement, reaming, graft sizing, graft implantation and fixation. BPTB and B-QT graft harvest is associated with increased risk of patella fracture. The fracture risk is increased in older patients with increased BMI, diabetes mellitus, osteoporosis, hypo-plastic patellae. Technically, non-trapezoidal cut geometry, deep cuts and cross-cutting edges have been shown to be associated with increased risk of patella fracture. Patella and tibial fractures may occur during surgery but are typically the result of relevant forces during rehabilitation. Displaced patellar fractures tend to undergo ORIF while undisplaced fractures may be treated conservatively. Assessment of patellar morphology is recommended when grafts with patellar bone blocks are to be used. Similarly, assessment of adequate insertional dimension is recommended prior to bundle ACLR. Grafts dropped during surgery can typically be implanted following relevant sterilisation with chlorhexidine. Premature hamstring graft amputation occurs primarily based on insufficient vinculae release. In these cases, tendon arms are folded to obtain an adequately sized graft with a minimal length of 5.5 cm. Saphenous nerve injury occurs primarily during skin incision for the infrapatellar branch and during tendon harvest for the terminal sartorial branch. Desensitisation techniques have shown to be associated with symptom improvement in most cases. Patellar tendon mismatch with a protruding tibial bone block may occur. Bone blocks can be shortened or the graft can be pulled higher into the femoral socket. Complications involving reaming comprise tunnel malpositioning, iatrogen structural damage, e.g. under-reaming the tibial plateau or eliminating the lateral posterior meniscal root [80, 81], as well as thermal damage, especially relevant in ACLR with open physes. A tibial tunnel placed too anteriorly induces notch impingement and mechanical graft failure. A tibial tunnel placed too posteriorly creates a short vertical graft construct with risk of PCL impingement and mechanical graft failure. A femoral tunnel placed anteriorly results in loss of flexion. A femoral tunnel placed too posteriorly may result in complete tunnel blow. Remaining in hyper-flexion is necessary to minimise the risk of tunnel blow out. In the case of significant tunnel blow out, revision drilling with an adequate trajectory is recommended and outside-in drilling may be considered. A femoral tunnel placed to vertical is typically associated with increased rotational laxity, eventually leading to graft failure. Graft screw divergence may occur if the screw is inserted in a different knee angle in which reaming was performed and may result in graft laceration or bone block amputation. In cases of bone-block amputation, the graft should be inspected for suitability and may be implanted as a pure tendon graft. Complications in the course of rehabilitation include one or two sided loss of motion, commonly treated with aggressive rehabilitation, manipulation under anaesthesia and/or lysis of adhesions. Septic arthritis following ACLR represents one of the most feared complications [50] and has an estimated incidence of approximately 1%. Acute infection (within the first two weeks) is commonly differentiated from subacute (between 2 weeks and 2 months) and chronic infection (more than 2 months postoperatively). Acute infection is commonly differentiated from low-virulent infection. Blood samples examining Leukocytes and CRP are typically obtained. Joint fluid aspiration is recommended [25, 179]. Cut-off values indicating surgery vary widely in the literature and range between 17.500 and 50.000/μl. High granulocyte concentrations (> 90%) are thought to be indicative of acute infection and are associated with increased risk of cartilage deterioration. Aggressive lavage is typically indicated in these cases [171]. Microbiological analysis including gram staining and culturing is recommended. During surgery, compromised tissue must be removed and an irrigation volume of 10–18 L of NaCl is recommended [50]. The ACL graft is typically retained in the primary intervention. If removed, culture examination of the graft is recommended. 3–5 representative tissue samples are obtained. Baker cysts should be considered as potential re-infection pathways. A reduced incidence of septic arthritis has been observed if ACL grafts are soaked in antibiotic solutions prior to implantation [145, 177]. Staphylococcus aureus and coagulase-negative staphylococci represent the most frequently found bacteria of underlying septic arthritis. Initial intravenous relevant antibiotic therapy for two weeks, followed by oral antibiotic therapy for further 5–6 weeks is typically recommended. The diagnosis of low-virulent infections represents a diagnostic challenge. Chronic pain, arthrofibrosis and increased activity around bone tunnels (as seen on MRI) are considered signs indicative of low-virulent infection.

## 13 Results of ACL Reconstruction

ACL reconstruction as a treatment strategy for ACL deficiency in the unselected population is commonly associated with satisfactory results. However, results are defined based on different measures including clinical measures of knee function [7], ACL-graft integrity [9], PROM´s as well as extent of adverse effects. To date, there is no universal definition of an acceptable result following ACL reconstruction as several factors including patient expectation play an important role. When compared to non-operative treatment, ACLR is associated with significantly superior short-term clinical and functional outcome [60]. However, the functional superiority of ACLR compared to nonoperative treatment of ACL deficiency does not translate to routine activities of daily living [60]. In addition, ACL reconstruction is not superior in terms of subjective outcomes, albeit the different nature of life-adapting mechanisms of both groups may represent a relevant bias [137]. Even though ACL reconstruction is thought to reduce the risk of irreparable meniscus and chondral injury in comparison to nonoperative treatment of ACL deficiency, ACLR does not reduce the risk of osteoarthritis [60]. In a recent meta-analysis with a mean long-term follow-up of 22.7 years following ACL reconstruction, Grassi et al. found that most patients showed satisfactory clinical subjective and objective outcomes as well as low revision and clinical failure rates of 7.9 and 4.5%, respectively. Abnormal laxity was observed in 10% of the cases, while OA was observed in 73% of the cases. Severe OA was observed in 12.8% of the cases and the overall TKA conversion rate was found to be 1.1% [47]. High demand athletes and delayed ACL reconstruction of more than 24 months following ACL injury were associated with higher TKA conversion rates. The significance of long-term clinical outcomes and resulting implications for current concepts is affected by the ongoing refinement of surgical techniques, hardware and rehabilitation concepts.

## References

1. Akazawa T, Miyamoto N, Nishio H, Miyamoto-Mikami E, Kinoshita M, Kobayashi Y, Nagao M, Takazawa Y. Age-related changes in mechanical properties of semitendinosus tendon used for anterior cruciate ligament reconstruction. J Orthop Surg Res 2022;17:501. https://doi.org/10.1186/s13018-022-03395-9
2. Alomar AZ, Alfayez SM, Somily AM. Hamstring autografts are associated with a high rate of contamination in anterior cruciate ligament reconstruction. Knee Surg Sports Traumatol Arthrosc. 2018;26(5):1357–61.
3. Amendola A, Menon M, Clatworthy M, Fowler PJ. The effect of fixation technique on graft position in anterior cruciate ligament reconstruction. Iowa Orthop J. 2003;23:29–35.
4. Anderson AF, Snyder RB, Lipscomb AB. Anterior cruciate ligament reconstruction. A prospective randomized study of three surgical methods. Am J Sports Med. 2001;29.
5. Araujo PH. Individualized ACL reconstruction. Knee Surg Sports Traumatol Arthrosc. 2014;22.

6. Ardern CL, Taylor NF, Feller JA, Whitehead TS, Webster KE. Psychological responses matter in returning to preinjury level of sport after anterior cruciate ligament reconstruction surgery. Am J Sports Med. 2013;41.
7. Ayeni OR. Pivot shift as an outcome measure for ACL reconstruction: a systematic review. Knee Surg Sports Traumatol Arthrosc. 2012;20.
8. Baawa-Ameyaw J, Plastow R, Begum F, Kayani B, Jeddy H, Haddad F. Current concepts in graft selection for anterior cruciate ligament reconstruction. EFORT Open Rev. 2021;6:808–15.
9. Barber-Westin S, Noyes FR. One in 5 athletes sustain reinjury upon return to high-risk sports after ACL reconstruction: a systematic review in 1239 athletes younger than 20 years. Sports Health. 2020;12(6):587–97.
10. Bernard M, Hertel P, Hornung H, Cierpinski T. Femoral insertion of the ACL. Radiographic quadrant method. Am J Knee Surg. 1997;10.
11. Beynnon BD, Johnson RJ, Abate JA, Fleming BC, Nichols CE. Treatment of anterior cruciate ligament injuries, part I. Am J Sports Med. 2005;33.
12. Bhattacharyya R, Ker A, Fogg Q, Spencer SJ, Joseph J. Lateral Intercondylar Ridge: Is it a reliable landmark for femoral ACL insertion?: An anatomical study. Int J Surg. 2018 Feb;50:55–59. https://doi.org/10.1016/j.ijsu.2017.12.013. Epub 2017 Dec 15. PMID: 29253556.
13. Blanke F, Trinnes K, Oehler N, Prall W, Lutter C, Tischer T, et al. Spontaneous healing of acute ACL ruptures: rate, prognostic factors and short-term outcome. Arch Orthop Trauma Surg. 2022;143:1–8.
14. Boden BP, Sheehan FT. Mechanism of non-contact ACL injury: OREF clinical research award 2021. J Orthop Res. 2022;40(3):531–40.
15. Boden BP, Breit I, Sheehan FT. Tibiofemoral alignment: contributing factors to noncontact anterior cruciate ligament injury. J Bone Joint Surg Am. 2009;91.
16. Boden BP, Dean GS, Feagin JA, Garrett WE. Mechanisms of anterior cruciate ligament injury. Orthopedics. 2000;23.
17. Brown CH Jr. Editorial commentary: how to increase hamstring tendon graft size for anterior cruciate ligament reconstruction. Arthroscopy. 2018;34(9):2641–6.
18. Brown CA, McAdams TR, Harris AHS, Maffulli C, Safran MR. ACL reconstruction in patients aged 40 years and older: a systematic review and introduction of a new Methodology Score for ACL studies. Am J Sports Med. 2013;41.
19. Cha PS, Brucker PU, West RV, Zelle BA, Yagi M, Kurosaka M. Arthroscopic double-bundle anterior cruciate ligament reconstruction: an anatomic approach. Arthroscopy. 2005;21.
20. Chambat P, Guier C, Sonnery-Cottet B, Fayard JM, Thaunat M. The evolution of ACL reconstruction over the last fifty years. Int Orthop. 2013;37.
21. Chen H, Chen B, Tie K, Fu Z, Chen L. Single-bundle versus double-bundle autologous anterior cruciate ligament reconstruction: a meta-analysis of randomized controlled trials at 5-year minimum follow-up. J Orthop Surg Res. 2018;13(1):50.
22. Christensen JJ, Krych AJ, Engasser WM, Vanhees MK, Collins MS, Dahm DL. Lateral tibial posterior slope is increased in patients with early graft failure after anterior cruciate ligament reconstruction. Am J Sports Med. 2015;43.
23. Clatworthy M, Sauer S, Roberts T. Transportal central femoral tunnel placement has a significantly higher revision rate than transtibial AM femoral tunnel placement in hamstring ACL reconstruction. Knee Surg Sports Traumatol Arthrosc 2019;27:124–129. https://doi.org/10.1007/s00167-018-5036-x
24. Colombet P, Dejour D, Panisset JC, Siebold R. Current concept of partial anterior cruciate ligament ruptures. Orthop Traumatol Surg Res. 2010;96.
25. Costa GG, Grassi A, Lo Presti M, Cialdella S, Zamparini E, Viale P, et al. White Blood cell count is the most reliable test for the diagnosis of septic arthritis after anterior cruciate ligament reconstruction: an observational study of 38 patients. Arthroscopy. 2021;37(5):1522-30.e2.
26. Costa GG, Grassi A, Perelli S, Agrò G, Bozzi F, Lo Presti M, et al. Age over 50 years is not a contraindication for anterior cruciate ligament reconstruction. Knee Surg Sports Traumatol Arthrosc. 2019;27(11):3679–91.

27. Darabos N, Haspl M, Moser C, Darabos A, Bartolek D, Groenemeyer D. Intraarticular application of autologous conditioned serum (ACS) reduces bone tunnel widening after ACL reconstructive surgery in a randomized controlled trial. Knee Surg Sports Traumatol Arthrosc. 2011 Dec;19 Suppl 1:S36-46. https://doi.org/10.1007/s00167-011-1458-4. Epub 2011 Mar 1. Erratum in: Knee Surg Sports Traumatol Arthrosc. 2019 Apr;27(4):1355. https://doi.org/10.1007/s00167-018-5222-x. PMID: 21360125.
28. DeMorat G, Weinhold P, Blackburn T, Chudik S, Garrett W. Aggressive quadriceps loading can induce noncontact anterior cruciate ligament injury. Am J Sports Med. 2004;32.
29. Dejour D, Pungitore M, Valluy J, Nover L, Saffarini M, Demey G. Preoperative laxity in ACL-deficient knees increases with posterior tibial slope and medial meniscal tears. Knee Surg Sports Traumatol Arthrosc. 2019;27(2):564–72.
30. Diek FM, Wolf MR, Murawski CD, Eck CF, Fu FH. Knee morphology and risk factors for developing an anterior cruciate ligament rupture: an MRI comparison between ACL-ruptured and non-injured knees. Knee Surg Sports Traumatol Arthrosc. 2014;22.
31. Dietvorst M, van der Steen MCM, Reijman M, Janssen RPA. Diagnostic values of history taking, physical examination and KT-1000 arthrometer for suspect anterior cruciate ligament injuries in children and adolescents: a prospective diagnostic study. BMC Musculoskelet Disord. 2022;23(1):710.
32. Eastlack ME, Axe MJ, Snyder-Mackler L. Laxity, instability, and functional outcome after ACL injury: copers versus noncopers. Med Sci Sports Exerc. 1999;31.
33. Ebert J, Edwards P, Annear P. Selective bundle reconstruction for symptomatic partial anterior cruciate ligament tears demonstrates good functional scores, high return to sport rates and a low re-tear rate. Knee. 2022;36:53–64.
34. Eck CF, Kropf EJ, Romanowski JR, Lesniak BP, Tranovich MJ, Dijk CN, et al. Factors that influence the intra-articular rupture pattern of the ACL graft following single bundle reconstruction. Knee Surg Sports Traumatol Arthrosc. 2011;19.
35. Eck CF, Limpisvasti O, ElAttrache NS. Is there a role for internal bracing and repair of the anterior cruciate ligament? A systematic literature review. Am J Sports Med. 2018;46.
36. Evans-Pickett A, Longobardi L, Spang JT, Creighton RA, Kamath G, Davis-Wilson HC, Loeser R, Blackburn JT, Pietrosimone B. Synovial fluid concentrations of matrix Metalloproteinase-3 and Interluekin-6 following anterior cruciate ligament injury associate with gait biomechanics 6 months following reconstruction. Osteoarthritis Cartilage. 2021 Jul;29(7):1006–1019. https://doi.org/10.1016/j.joca.2021.03.014. Epub 2021 Mar 27. PMID: 33781899; PMCID: PMC8658576.
37. Favian Ding Jie Ng, Denny Tjiauw Tjoen Lie, Andy Yew, Relooking at double-bundle versus single-bundle anterior cruciate ligament reconstruction: A biomechanical model to evaluate which can confer better rotatory stability. Clinical Biomechanics. 2022;99:105758, ISSN 0268-0033. https://doi.org/10.1016/j.clinbiomech.2022.105758.
38. Ferretti A, Carrozzo A, Saithna A, Argento G, Annibaldi A, Latini F, et al. Comparison of primary repair of the anterior cruciate ligament and anterolateral structures to reconstruction and lateral extra-articular Tenodesis at 2-year follow-up. Am J Sports Med. 2023;51(9):2300–12.
39. Feucht MJ, Mauro CS, Brucker PU, Imhoff AB, Hinterwimmer S. The role of the tibial slope in sustaining and treating anterior cruciate ligament injuries. Knee Surg Sports Traumatol Arthrosc. 2013;21.
40. Figueroa F, Figueroa D, Espregueira-Mendes J. Hamstring autograft size importance in anterior cruciate ligament repair surgery. EFORT Open Rev. 2018;3(3):93–7.
41. Fritsch B, Figueroa F, Semay B. Graft preparation technique to optimize hamstring graft diameter for anterior cruciate ligament reconstruction. Arthrosc Tech. 2017;6.
42. Fu FH, Bennett CH, Lattermann C, Ma CB. Current trends in anterior cruciate ligament reconstruction. Part 1: Biology and biomechanics of reconstruction. Am J Sports Med. 1999;27.
43. Gao F, Zhou J, He C, Ding J, Lou Z, Xie Q, et al. A morphologic and quantitative study of mechanoreceptors in the remnant stump of the human anterior cruciate ligament. Arthroscopy. 2016;32.

44. Georgiev GP, Telang M, Landzhov B, Olewnik Ł, Slavchev SA, LaPrade RF, et al. The novel epiligament theory: differences in healing failure between the medial collateral and anterior cruciate ligaments. J Exp Orthop. 2022;9(1):10.
45. Georgiev G, Yordanov Y, Olewnik Ł, Tubbs R, LaPrade R, Ananiev J, et al. Do the differences in the epiligament of the proximal and distal parts of the anterior cruciate ligament explain their different healing capacities? Quantitative and immunohistochemical analysis of CD34 and α-SMA expression in relation to the epiligament theory. Biomedicines. 2024;12:156.
46. Girgis FG, Marshall JL, Monajem A. The cruciate ligaments of the knee joint. Anatomical, functional and experimental analysis. Clin Orthop Relat Res. 1975;106.
47. Grassi A, Agostinone P, Di Paolo S, Lucidi GA, Macchiarola L, Bontempi M, et al. Knee position at the moment of bone bruise could reflect the late phase of non-contact anterior cruciate ligament injury rather than the mechanisms leading to ligament failure. Knee Surg Sports Traumatol Arthrosc. 2021;29(12):4138–45.
48. Grood ES, Suntay WJ. A joint coordinate system for the clinical description of three-dimensional motions: application to the knee. J Biomech Eng. 1983;105.
49. Guimarães TM, Giglio PN, Sobrado MF, Bonadio MB, Gobbi RG, Pécora JR, et al. Knee hyperextension greater than 5° is a risk factor for failure in ACL reconstruction using hamstring graft. Orthop J Sports Med. 2021;9(11):23259671211056324.
50. Gupta R, Sood M, Malhotra A, Masih GD, Raghav M, Khanna T. Incidence, risk factors, and management of infection following anterior cruciate ligament reconstruction surgery. Indian J Orthop. 2018;52(4):399–405.
51. Hamner DL, Brown CH Jr, Steiner ME, Hecker AT, Hayes WC. Hamstring tendon grafts for reconstruction of the anterior cruciate ligament: biomechanical evaluation of the use of multiple strands and tensioning techniques. J Bone Joint Surg Am. 1999;81(4):549–57.
52. Hashemi J, Breighner R, Chandrashekar N, Hardy DM, Chaudhari AM, Shultz SJ, et al. Hip extension, knee flexion paradox: a new mechanism for non-contact ACL injury. J Biomech. 2011;44.
53. Hashemi J, Chandrashekar N, Gill B, Beynnon BD, Slauterbeck JR, Schutt RC, et al. The geometry of the tibial plateau and its influence on the biomechanics of the tibiofemoral joint. J Bone Jt Surg Am. 2008;90.
54. Hashemi J, Chandrashekar N, Mansouri H, Gill B, Slauterbeck JR, Schutt RC, et al. Shallow medial tibial plateau and steep medial and lateral tibial slopes: new risk factors for anterior cruciate ligament injuries. Am J Sports Med. 2010;38.
55. Hashemi J, Breighner R, Chandrashekar N, Hardy DM, Chaudhari AM, Shultz SJ, et al. Hip extension, knee flexion paradox: A new mechanism for non-contact ACL injury. J Biomech. 2011;44(4):577–85.
56. Haupt E, KJ OK, Clay TB, Kenney N, Farmer KW. Biomechanical Properties of Small-Size Hamstring Autografts. Cureus. 2020;12(6):e8728.
57. Hefzy MS, Grood ES, Noyes FR. Factors affecting the region of most isometric femoral attachments. Part II: the anterior cruciate ligament. Am J Sports Med. 1989;17.
58. Hewett TE, Myer GD, Zazulak BT. Hamstrings to quadriceps peak torque ratios diverge between sexes with increasing isokinetic angular velocity. J Sci Med Sport. 2008;11.
59. Hohmann E, Bryant A, Reaburn P, Tetsworth K. Is there a correlation between posterior tibial slope and non-contact anterior cruciate ligament injuries? Knee Surg Sports Traumatol Arthrosc. 2011;19.
60. Hohmann E, Tetsworth K, Glatt V. Anterior cruciate ligament reconstruction results in better patient reported outcomes but has no advantage for activities of daily living or the subsequent development of osteoarthritis. A systematic review and meta-analysis. The Knee. 2023;41:137–49.
61. Hoshino Y. In Vivo Measurement of the Pivot-Shift Test in the Anterior Cruciate Ligament–Deficient Knee Using an Electromagnetic Device. Am J Sports Med. 2007;35.
62. Hoshino Y. Quantitative evaluation of the pivot shift by image analysis using the iPad. Knee Surg Sports Traumatol Arthrosc. 2013;21.

63. Hoshino Y, Nagamune K, Yagi M, Araki D, Nishimoto K, Kubo S. The effect of intra-operative knee flexion angle on determination of graft location in the anatomic double-bundle anterior cruciate ligament reconstruction. Knee Surg Sports Traumatol Arthrosc. 2009;17.
64. Hoshino Y, Rothrauff BB, Hensler D, Fu FH, Musahl V. Arthroscopic image distortion-part I: the effect of lens and viewing angles in a 2-dimensional in vitro model. Knee Surg Sports Traumatol Arthrosc. 2014.
65. Hoshino Y, Rothrauff BB, Hensler D, Fu FH, Musahl V. Arthroscopic image distortion-part II: the effect of lens angle and portal location in a 3D knee model. Knee Surg Sports Traumatol Arthrosc. 2014.
66. Hudek R, Fuchs B, Regenfelder F, Koch PP. Is noncontact ACL injury associated with the posterior tibial and meniscal slope? Clin Orthop Relat Res. 2011;469.
67. Iio K, Tsuda E, Tsukada H, Yamamoto Y, Maeda S, Naraoka T, et al. Characteristics of elongated and ruptured anterior cruciate ligament grafts: An analysis of 21 consecutive revision cases. Asia-Pacific J Sports Med Arthrosc Rehabil Technol. 2017;8:1–7.
68. Inderhaug E, Larsen A, Waaler PA, Strand T, Harlem T, Solheim E. The effect of intraoperative fluoroscopy on the accuracy of femoral tunnel placement in single-bundle anatomic ACL reconstruction. Knee Surg Sports Traumatol Arthrosc. 2017;25.
69. James EW, Dawkins BJ, Schachne JM, Ganley TJ, Kocher MS, Anderson CN, et al. Early operative versus delayed operative versus nonoperative treatment of pediatric and adolescent anterior cruciate ligament injuries: a systematic review and meta-analysis. Am J Sports Med. 2021;49(14):4008–17.
70. Järvelä T, Nurmi Janne T, Järvelä S. Anatomic double-bundle anterior cruciate ligament reconstruction using soft tissue interference screw fixation. Annals of Joint. 2018;3. https://aoj.amegroups.org/article/view/4723
71. Kassam A-A, Tillotson L, Schranz P, Mandalia V. The lateral meniscus as a guide to anatomical Tibial tunnel placement during anterior cruciate ligament reconstruction. Open Orthopaed J. 2015;9:542–7.
72. Katagiri H, Nakamura K, Muneta T, Watanabe T, Miyatake K, Sekiya I, et al. Inflammatory and healing environment in synovial fluid after anterior cruciate ligament reconstruction: granulocytes and endogenous opioids as new targets of postoperative pain. Biochem Biophys Rep. 2021;26:100981.
73. Kato Y, Ingham SJ, Kramer S, Smolinski P, Saito A, Fu FH. Effect of tunnel position for anatomic single-bundle ACL reconstruction on knee biomechanics in a porcine model. Knee Surg Sports Traumatol Arthrosc. 2010;18.
74. Kim J, Baek S, Schlecht S, Beaulieu M, Bussau L, Chen J, et al. Anterior cruciate ligament microfatigue damage detected by collagen autofluorescence in situ. J Exp Orthopaed. 2022;9.
75. Koga H, Muneta T, Yagishita K, Ju YJ, Sekiya I. The effect of graft fixation angles on anteroposterior and rotational knee laxity in double-bundle anterior cruciate ligament reconstruction: evaluation using computerized navigation. Am J Sports Med. 2012;40(3):615–23.
76. Koga H, Nakamae A, Shima Y, Iwasa J, Myklebust G, Engebretsen L, et al. Mechanisms for noncontact anterior cruciate ligament injuries: knee joint kinematics in 10 injury situations from female team handball and basketball. Am J Sports Med. 2010;38.
77. Kopf S, Kauert R, Halfpaap J, Jung T, Becker R. A new quantitative method for pivot shift grading. Knee Surg Sports Traumatol Arthrosc. 2012;20(4):718–23.
78. Kruppa P, Flies A, Wulsten D, Collette R, Duda G, Schaser K-D, et al. Significant loss of ACL graft force with Tibial-sided soft tissue interference screw fixation over 24 hours: a biomechanical study. Orthop J Sports Med. 2020;8:232596712091643.
79. Kvist J, Kartus J, Karlsson J, Forssblad M. Results from the Swedish national anterior cruciate ligament register. Arthroscopy. 2014;30.
80. LaPrade CM, Jisa KA, Cram TR, LaPrade RF. Posterior lateral meniscal root tear due to a malpositioned double-bundle anterior cruciate ligament reconstruction tibial tunnel. Knee Surg Sports Traumatol Arthrosc. 2014.
81. LaPrade CM, Smith SD, Rasmussen MT, Hamming MG, Wijdicks CA, Engebretsen L. Consequences of tibial tunnel reaming on the meniscal roots during cruciate ligament reconstruction in a cadaveric model, part 1: the anterior cruciate ligament. Am J Sports Med. 2015;43.

82. Lattermann C, Conley CE, Johnson DL, Reinke EK, Huston LJ, Huebner JL, Chou CH, Kraus VB, Spindler KP, Jacobs CA. Select Biomarkers on the Day of Anterior Cruciate Ligament Reconstruction Predict Poor Patient-Reported Outcomes at 2-Year Follow-Up: A Pilot Study. Biomed Res Int. 2018 Jul 19;2018:9387809. https://doi.org/10.1155/2018/9387809. PMID: 30105266; PMCID: PMC6076965.
83. Legler J, Laverdiere C, Boily M, Tarchala M, Hart A, Martineau PA. Evaluating femoral graft placement using three-dimensional magnetic resonance imaging in the reconstruction of the anterior cruciate ligament via independent or transtibial drilling techniques: a retrospective cohort study. Eur J Orthopaed Surg Traumatol. 2023.
84. Levy IM, Torzilli PA, Warren RF. The effect of medial meniscectomy on anterior-posterior motion of the knee. J Bone Joint Surg Am. 1982;64.
85. Li Y, Hong L, Feng H, Wang Q, Zhang J, Song G, et al. Posterior Tibial slope influences static anterior Tibial translation in anterior cruciate ligament reconstruction: a minimum 2-year follow-up study. Am J Sports Med. 2014;42(4):927–33.
86. Lin L, Wang H, Wang J, Wang Y, Chen Y, Yu J-K. Effects of higher femoral tunnels on clinical outcomes, MRI, and second-look findings in double-bundle anterior cruciate ligament reconstruction with a minimal 5-year follow-up. Chin Med J. 2024.
87. Liu A, Cui W, Yang W, Li C, Yan S, Xin Z, et al. Anterior tibial subluxation of lateral compartment is associated with high-grade rotatory instability for acute but not chronic anterior cruciate ligament injuries: an MRI case-control study. Arthrosc J Arthrosc Relat Surg. 2022;38.
88. Lopomo N. Quantitative assessment of pivot-shift using inertial sensors. Knee Surg Sports Traumatol Arthrosc. 2012;20.
89. Lopomo N, Zaffagnini S, Amis AA. Quantifying the pivot shift test: a systematic review. Knee Surg Sports Traumatol Arthrosc. 2013;21.
90. Luites JWH, Wymenga AB, Blankevoort L, Kooloos JGM. Description of the attachment geometry of the anteromedial and posterolateral bundles of the ACL from arthroscopic perspecti for anatomical tunnel placement.Knee Surg Sports Traumatol Arthrosc. 2007;15(12):1422–31. https://doi.org/10.1007/s00167-007-0402-0
91. MacWilliams BA, Wilson DR, DesJardins JD, Romero J, Chao EY. Hamstrings cocontraction reduces internal rotation, anterior translation, and anterior cruciate ligament load in weight-bearing flexion. J Orthop Res. 1999;17.
92. Magnussen RA, Lawrence JT, West RL, Toth AP, Taylor DC, Garrett WE. Graft size and patient age are predictors of early revision after anterior cruciate ligament reconstruction with hamstring autograft. Arthroscopy. 2012;28(4):526–31.
93. Magnussen RA, Reinke EK, Huston LJ, Hewett TE, Spindler KP. Factors associated with high-grade lachman, pivot shift, and anterior drawer at the time of anterior cruciate ligament reconstruction. Arthroscopy. 2016;32.
94. Mall NA, Chalmers PN, Moric M, Tanaka MJ, Cole BJ, Bach BR, et al. Incidence and trends of anterior cruciate ligament reconstruction in the United States. Am J Sports Med. 2014;42.
95. Mandelbaum BR, Silvers HJ, Watanabe DS, Knarr JF, Thomas SD, Griffin LY, et al. Effectiveness of a neuromuscular and proprioceptive training program in preventing anterior cruciate ligament injuries in female athletes: 2-year follow-up. Am J Sports Med. 2005;33.
96. Mariscalco MW, Flanigan DC, Mitchell J, Pedroza AD, Jones MH, Andrish JT, et al. The influence of hamstring autograft size on patient-reported outcomes and risk of revision after anterior cruciate ligament reconstruction: a multicenter orthopaedic outcomes network (MOON) Cohort Study. Arthroscopy. 2013;29(12):1948–53.
97. Matsumoto Y, Takahashi T, Hatayama K, Kubo T, Higuchi H, Kimura M, et al. Arthrosc Sports Med Rehabil. 2021;3(6):e1967–73.
98. Matsumoto H. Mechanism of the pivot shift. J Bone Joint Surg Br. 1990;72.
99. McConkey MO, Amendola A, Ramme AJ, Dunn WR, Flanigan DC, Britton CL, et al. Arthroscopic agreement among surgeons on anterior cruciate ligament tunnel placement. Am J Sports Med. 2012;40.

100. McLean SG, Lucey SM, Rohrer S, Brandon C. Knee joint anatomy predicts high-risk in vivo dynamic landing knee biomechanics. Clin Biomech (Bristol, Avon). 2010;25.
101. McLean SG, Oh YK, Palmer ML, Lucey SM, Lucarelli DG, Ashton-Miller JA, et al. The relationship between anterior tibial acceleration, tibial slope, and ACL strain during a simulated jump landing task. J Bone Jt Surg Am. 2011;93.
102. de Mees TTCR, Reijman M, Waarsing JH, Meuffels DE. Posteriorly positioned femoral grafts decrease long-term failure in anterior cruciate ligament reconstruction, femoral and tibial graft positions did not affect long-term reported outcome. Knee Surg Sports Traumatol Arthrosc. 2022;30(6):2003–13.
103. Meyer EG, Haut RC. Excessive compression of the human tibio-femoral joint causes ACL rupture. J Biomech. 2005;38(11):2311–6.
104. Michel E, Jordan E, Canovas F, Bouchdoug K, Dagneaux L, Gaillard F. Influence of residual anterior laxity on functional outcomes after anterior cruciate ligament reconstruction. Orthop Traumatol Surg Res. 2022;108:103264.
105. Moloney G, Araujo P, Rabuck S, Carey R, Rincon G, Zhang X, et al. Use of a fluoroscopic overlay to assist arthroscopic anterior cruciate ligament reconstruction. Am J Sports Med. 2013;41.
106. Moran J, LaPrade R, Medvecky M. Examining the distribution of bone bruise patterns in contact and noncontact acute anterior cruciate ligament injuries: response. Am J Sports Med. 2023;51.
107. Murgier J, Powell A, Young S, Clatworthy M. Effectiveness of thicker hamstring or patella tendon grafts to reduce graft failure rate in anterior cruciate ligament reconstruction in young patients. Knee Surg Sports Traumatol Arthrosc. 2021;29(3):725–31.
108. Muro S, Kim J, Tsukada S, Akita K. Significance of the broad non-bony attachments of the anterior cruciate ligament on the tibial side. Sci Rep. 2022;12(1):6844.
109. Musahl V, Burkart A, Debski RE, Scyoc A, Fu FH, Woo SL. Anterior cruciate ligament tunnel placement: comparison of insertion site anatomy with the guidelines of a computer-assisted surgical system. Arthroscopy. 2003;19.
110. Musahl V, Voos J, O'Loughlin PF, Stueber V, Kendoff D, Pearle AD. Mechanized pivot shift test achieves greater accuracy than manual pivot shift test. Knee Surg Sports Traumatol Arthrosc Off J ESSKA. 2010;18.
111. Musahl V. Current trends in the anterior cruciate ligament part 1: biology and biomechanics. 2021.
112. Musgrove TP, Salmon LJ, Burt CF, Pinczewski LA. The influence of reverse-thread screw femoral fixation on laxity measurements after anterior cruciate ligament reconstruction with hamstring tendon. Am J Sports Med. 2000;28(5):695–9.
113. Nakano N, Bartlett J, Khanduja V. Is restricted hip movement a risk factor for anterior cruciate ligament injury? J Orthop Surg. 2018;26(3):2309499018799520.
114. Nawabi D, Imhauser C, Tucker S, Nguyen J, Wickiewicz T, Pearle A. ACL fibers inserting on the lateral intercondylar ridge carry the greatest loads—are modern anatomic femoral tunnel positions too low? Orthopaed J Sports Med 2014;2.
115. Nebelung W, Becker R, Merkel M, Röpke M. Bone tunnel enlargement after anterior cruciate ligament reconstruction with semitendinosus tendon using Endobutton fixation on the femoral side. Arthroscopy 1998;14:810–5. https://doi.org/10.1016/s0749-8063(98)70015-5
116. Ng, Wing Hung Alex, Griffith, James Francis, Hung, Esther Hiu Yee, Paunipagar, Bhawan, Law, Billy Kan Yip & Yung, Patrick Shu Hang. Imaging of the anterior cruciate ligament. World journal of orthopedics 2011;2:75–84. doi: 10.5312/wjo.v2.i8.75. http://europepmc.org/abstract/MED/22474639 https://doi.org/10.5312/wjo.v2.i8.75 https://www.ncbi.nlm.nih.gov/pmc/articles/pmid/22474639/?tool=EBI https://www.ncbi.nlm.nih.gov/pmc/articles/pmid/22474639/pdf/?tool=EBI https://europepmc.org/articles/PMC3302044 https://europepmc.org/articles/PMC3302044?pdf=render
117. Noyes FR, Barber SD. The effect of an extra-articular procedure on allograft reconstructions for chronic ruptures of the anterior cruciate ligament. J Bone Joint Surg Am. 1991;73.

118. Noyes FR, Grood ES. The scientific basis for examination and classification of knee ligament injuries. Noyes' knee disorders: surgery, rehabilitation, clinical outcomes. Philadelphia: Elsevier; 2017.
119. Noyes FR, Huser LE, Jurgensmeier D, Walsh J, Levy MS. Is an anterolateral ligament reconstruction required in ACL-reconstructed knees with associated injury to the anterolateral structures? Am J Sports Med. 2017;45.
120. Noyes FR, Huser LE, Levy MS. Rotational knee instability in ACL-deficient knees: role of the anterolateral ligament and iliotibial band as defined by tibiofemoral compartment translations and rotations. J Bone Joint Surg Am. 2017;99.
121. O'Connor JJ. Can muscle co-contraction protect knee ligaments after injury or repair? J Bone Joint Surg Br. 1993;75.
122. O'Neill BJ, Byrne FJ, Hirpara KM, Brennan WF, McHugh PE, Curtin W. Anterior cruciate ligament graft tensioning. Is the maximal sustained one-handed pull technique reproducible? BMC Res Notes. 2011;4:244.
123. Oh, Jin-Young, Kim, Kun-Tae, Park, Young-Jin, Won, Hee-Chan, Yoo, Jun-Il, Moon, Dong-Kyu, Cho, Sung-Hee, Hwang, Sun-Chul. Biomechanical comparison of single-bundle versus double-bundle anterior cruciate ligament reconstruction: a meta-analysis. Knee Surgery & Related Research 2020;32:14. https://doi.org/10.1186/s43019-020-00033-8
124. Olsen OE, Myklebust G, Engebretsen L, Bahr R. Injury mechanisms for anterior cruciate ligament injuries in team handball: a systematic video analysis. Am J Sports Med. 2004;32.
125. Olsen OE, Myklebust G, Engebretsen L, Holme I, Bahr R. Relationship between floor type and risk of ACL injury in team handball. Scand J Med Sci Sports. 2003;13.
126. Onor G, Johns W, Patel N, Wilson S, Cook R, Ciccotti M, et al. Reconstruction vs. repair: a review of recent trends and controversies for management of ACL rupture. Current Orthopaedic Practice. 2023;35.
127. Pasanen K, Parkkari J, Rossi L, Kannus P. Artificial playing surface increases the injury risk in pivoting indoor sports: a prospective one-season follow-up study in Finnish female floorball. Br J Sports Med. 2008;42.
128. Pernin J, Verdonk P, Si Selmi TA, Massin P, Neyret P. Long-term follow-up of 24.5 years after intra-articular anterior cruciate ligament reconstruction with lateral extra-articular augmentation. Am J Sports Med. 2010;38.
129. Perry A, Knapik D, Maheshwer B, Polce E, Hodakowski A, Jackson G, et al. Lateral meniscus posterior root repair in the setting of anterior cruciate ligament reconstruction restores joint mechanics to the intact state and improves clinical function: a systematic review of biomechanical and clinical outcomes. Knee Surg Sports Traumatol Arthrosc. 2023;31.
130. Pfeiffer RP, Shea KG, Roberts D, Grandstrand S, Bond L. Lack of effect of a knee ligament injury prevention program on the incidence of noncontact anterior cruciate ligament injury. J Bone Joint Surg Am. 2006;88.
131. Phadke R, Song B. Effect of Graft Fixation Angles in Double-Bundle Anterior Cruciate Ligament Reconstruction, A Systematic Review; 2023.
132. Poehling-Monaghan KL, Salem H, Ross KE, Secrist E, Ciccotti MC, Tjoumakaris F, et al. Long-term outcomes in anterior cruciate ligament reconstruction: a systematic review of patellar tendon versus hamstring autografts. Orthop J Sports Med. 2017;5(6):2325967117709735.
133. Prodromidis AD, Drosatou C, Thivaios GC, Zreik N, Charalambous CP. Timing of anterior cruciate ligament reconstruction and relationship with meniscal tears: a systematic review and meta-analysis. Am J Sports Med. 2020;9.
134. Prodromos CC, Han Y, Rogowski J, Joyce B, Shi K. A meta-analysis of the incidence of anterior cruciate ligament tears as a function of gender, sport, and a knee injury-reduction regimen. Arthroscopy. 2007;23.
135. Ro DH, Han H-S, Lee MC. What has been learned in anterior cruciate ligament reconstruction during the past 20 years? J Korean Orthopaed Assoc. 2021;56:1.
136. Robinson JD Jr, Williamson T, Carson T, Whelan RJ, Abelow SP, Gilmer BB. Primary anterior cruciate ligament repair: Current concepts. J ISAKOS. 2023;8(6):456–66.

137. Rodriguez K, Soni M, Joshi PK, Patel SC, Shreya D, Zamora DI, et al. Anterior cruciate ligament injury: conservative versus surgical treatment. Cureus. 2021;13(12):e20206.
138. Rothrauff BB, Jorge A, Sa D, Kay J, Fu FH, Musahl V. Anatomic ACL reconstruction reduces risk of post-traumatic osteoarthritis: a systematic review with minimum 10-year follow-up. Knee Surg Sports Traumatol Arthrosc. 2019.
139. Runer A, Keeling L, Wagala N, Nugraha H, Özbek E, Hughes J, et al. Current trends in graft choice for anterior cruciate ligament reconstruction—Part I: anatomy, biomechanics, graft incorporation and fixation. J Exp Orthopaed. 2023;10:37.
140. Runer A, Csapo R, Hepperger C, Herbort M, Hoser C, Fink C. Anterior cruciate ligament reconstructions with quadriceps tendon autograft result in lower graft rupture rates but similar patient-reported outcomes as compared with hamstring tendon autograft: a comparison of 875 patients. Am J Sports Med. 2020;48.
141. Runer A. Current trends in graft choice for primary anterior cruciate ligament reconstruction – part II: In-vivo kinematics, patient reported outcomes, re-rupture rates, strength recovery, return to sports and complications. 2023.
142. Samitier G, Marcano A, Alentorn-Geli E, Cugat R, Farmer K, Moser M. Failure of anterior cruciate ligament reconstruction. Arch Bone Joint Surg. 2015;3:220–40.
143. Santos CF, Bastos R, Andrade R, Pereira R, Parente MPL, Jorge RN, et al. Revisiting the role of knee external rotation in non-contact ACL mechanism of injury. Appl Sci. 2023;13(6):3802.
144. Schimoler Patrick J, Braun David T, Miller Mark C, Akhavan S. Quadrupled Hamstring Graft Strength as a Function of Clinical Sizing. Arthroscopy: The Journal of Arthroscopic & Related Surgery 2015;31:1091–1096. https://doi.org/10.1016/j.arthro.2015.01.013, https://www.sciencedirect.com/science/article/pii/S0749806315000705
145. Schuster P, Schlumberger M, Mayer P, Eichinger M, Geßlein M, Richter J. Soaking of autografts in vancomycin is highly effective in preventing postoperative septic arthritis after revision anterior cruciate ligament reconstruction. Knee Surg Sports Traumatol Arthrosc. 2020;28(4):1154–8.
146. Selim NM. Anatomic Double-Bundle Anterior Cruciate Ligament Reconstruction with Hamstring Tendon Autograft through Single Femoral Tunnel and Single Branched Tibial Tunnel. Arthrosc Tech. 2018 Sep 10;7(10):e989–98. https://doi.org/10.1016/j.eats.2018.06.004. PMID: 30377578; PMCID: PMC6203690.
147. Seo S-S, Kim C-W, Lee C-R, Park D-H, Kwon Y-U, Kim O-G, et al. Intraoperative fluoroscopy reduces the variability in femoral tunnel placement during single-bundle anterior cruciate ligament reconstruction. Knee Surg Sports Traumatol Arthrosc. 2020;28(2):629–36.
148. Sgardelis P, Naqvi G, Servant C. Minimally invasive bone-patellar tendon-bone graft harvest is associated with less frequent anterior knee pain at rest than hamstring graft harvest after anterior cruciate ligament reconstruction at the 1-year follow-up. Arthrosc Sports Med Rehabil. 2023;5:100766.
149. Shelbourne KD, Roberson TA, Gray T. Long-term evaluation of posterior lateral meniscus root tears left in situ at the time of anterior cruciate ligament reconstruction. Am J Sports Med. 2011;39(7):1439–43.
150. Shelbourne KD, Wilckens JH, Mollabashy A, DeCarlo M. Arthrofibrosis in acute anterior cruciate ligament reconstruction. The effect of timing of reconstruction and rehabilitation. Am J Sports Med. 1991;19.
151. Shin CS, Chaudhari AM, Andriacchi TP. Valgus plus internal rotation moments increase anterior cruciate ligament strain more than either alone. Med Sci Sports Exerc. 2011;43.
152. Siegel L, Vandenakker-Albanese C, Siegel D. Anterior cruciate ligament injuries: anatomy, physiology, biomechanics, and management. Clin J Sport Med Off J Can Acad Sport Med. 2012;22:349–55.
153. Song GY, Zhang H, Zhang J, Liu X, Xue Z, Qian Y, et al. Greater static anterior tibial subluxation of the lateral compartment after an acute anterior cruciate ligament injury is associated with an increased posterior tibial slope. Am J Sports Med. 2018;46(7):1617–23.
154. Sonnery-Cottet B, Hopper GP, Gousopoulos L, Vieira TD, Thaunat M, Fayard J-M, et al. Arthrogenic muscle inhibition following knee injury or surgery: pathophysiology, classification, and treatment. Video J Sports Med. 2022;2(3):26350254221086296.

155. Sonnery-Cottet B, Archbold P, Cucurulo T, Fayard JM, Bortolletto J, Thaunat M, et al. The influence of the tibial slope and the size of the intercondylar notch on rupture of the anterior cruciate ligament. J Bone Jt Surg Br. 2011;93.
156. Sonnery-Cottet B, Lavoie F, Ogassawara R, Scussiato RG, Kidder JF, Chambat P. Selective anteromedial bundle reconstruction in partial ACL tears: a series of 36 patients with mean 24 months follow-up. Knee Surg Sports Traumatol Arthrosc. 2010;18.
157. Steffen K, Andersen TE, Bahr R. Risk of injury on artificial turf and natural grass in young female football players. Br J Sports Med. 2007;41.
158. Stephen JM, Halewood C, Kittl C, Bollen SR, Williams A, Amis AA. Posteromedial meniscocapsular lesions increase tibiofemoral joint laxity with anterior cruciate ligament deficiency, and their repair reduces laxity. Am J Sports Med. 2016;44.
159. Sullivan B, Stone AV, Conley CEW, Hunt ER, Lattermann C, Jacobs CA. Human synovial fluid interleukin-6, but not type II collagen breakdown, positively correlated with pain after anterior cruciate ligament injury and reconstruction. J Orthop Res. 2023;41(2):300–6.
160. Sundemo D, Senorski EH, Karlsson L, Horvath A, Juul-Kristensen B, Karlsson J, et al. Generalised joint hypermobility increases ACL injury risk and is associated with inferior outcome after ACL reconstruction: a systematic review. BMJ Open Sport Exerc Med. 2019;5(1):e000620.
161. Svantesson E, Hamrin Senorski E, Webster KE, Karlsson J, Diermeier T, Rothrauff BB, et al. Clinical outcomes after anterior cruciate ligament injury: panther symposium ACL injury clinical outcomes consensus group. J ISAKOS. 2020;5(5):281–94.
162. Svantesson E, Hamrin Senorski E, Östergaard M, Grassi A, Krupic F, Westin O, et al. Graft choice for anterior cruciate ligament reconstruction with a concomitant non-surgically treated medial collateral ligament injury does not influence the risk of revision. Arthroscopy. 2020;36(1):199–211.
163. Sven S, Maurice B, Hoeher J, Marc B. Variability of tunnel positioning in fluoroscopic-assisted ACL reconstruction. Knee Surg Sports Traumatol Arthrosc. 2015;23.
164. Tegner Y, Lysholm J. Rating systems in the evaluation of knee ligament injuries. Clin Orthop Relat Res. 1985;198.
165. Thaunat M, Fayard JM, Guimaraes TM, Jan N, Murphy CG, Sonnery-Cottet B. Classification and surgical repair of ramp lesions of the medial meniscus. Arthrosc Tech. 2016;5(4):e871–5.
166. Thompson S, Salmon L, Waller A, Linklater J, Roe J, Pinczewski L. Twenty-year outcomes of a longitudinal prospective evaluation of isolated endoscopic anterior cruciate ligament reconstruction with patellar tendon autografts. Am J Sports Med. 2015;43.
167. Thürig G, Panadero-Morales R, Giovannelli L, Kocher F, Peris JL, Tannast M, Petek D. Compressed Lateral and anteroposterior Anatomical Systematic Sequences «CLASS»: compressed MRI sequences with assessed anatomical femoral and tibial ACL's footprints, a feasibility study. J Exp Orthop 2022;9:8. https://doi.org/10.1186/s40634-022-00445-3
168. Tischer T, Beaufilis P, Becker R, Ahmad S, Bonomo M, Dejour D, et al. Management of anterior cruciate ligament revision in adults: the 2022 ESSKA consensus part I-diagnostics and preoperative planning. Knee Surg Sports Traumatol Arthrosc. 2022;31.
169. Tjoumakaris FP, Herz-Brown AL, Bowers AL, Sennett BJ, Bernstein J. Complications in brief: anterior cruciate ligament reconstruction. Clin Orthop Relat Res. 2012;470(2):630–6.
170. Tjoumakaris FP, Donegan DJ, Sekiya JK. Partial tears of the anterior cruciate ligament: Diagnosis and treatment. Am J Orthoped. 2011;40.
171. Torres-Claramunt R, Pelfort X, Erquicia J, Gil-González S, Gelber PE, Puig L, et al. Knee joint infection after ACL reconstruction: prevalence, management and functional outcomes. Knee Surg Sports Traumatol Arthrosc. 2013;21(12):2844–9.
172. Tuca M, Valderrama I, Eriksson K, Tapasvi S. Current trends in anterior cruciate ligament surgery. A worldwide benchmark study. J isakos 2023;8:2–10. https://doi.org/10.1016/j.jisako.2022.08.009
173. Tuman JM, Diduch DR, Rubino LJ, Baumfeld JA, Nguyen HS, Hart JM. Predictors for hamstring graft diameter in anterior cruciate ligament reconstruction. Am J Sports Med. 2007;35(11):1945–9.

174. Utzschneider S, Goettinger M, Weber P, Horng A, Glaser C, Jansson V, et al. Development and validation of a new method for the radiologic measurement of the tibial slope. Knee Surg Sports Traumatol Arthrosc. 2011;19.
175. Vaishya R, Hasija R. Joint Hypermobility and Anterior Cruciate Ligament Injury. J Orthop Surg. 2013;21(2):182–4.
176. Vari N, Marot V, Cavaignac M, Vieira T, Bérard É, Cavaignac E. Factors affecting graft remodeling and anterior cruciate ligament reconstruction: MRI study of 180 knees. Am J Sports Med. 2023;51:3635465231171947.
177. Vertullo CJ, Quick M, Jones A, Grayson JE. A surgical technique using presoaked vancomycin hamstring grafts to decrease the risk of infection after anterior cruciate ligament reconstruction. Arthroscopy. 2012;28(3):337–42.
178. Voos JE, Musahl V, Maak TG, Wickiewicz TL, Pearle AD. Comparison of tunnel positions in single-bundle anterior cruciate ligament reconstructions using computer navigation. Knee Surg, Sports Traumatol, Arthrosc: Off J ESSKA. 2010;18.
179. Wang C, Lee YHD, Siebold R. Recommendations for the management of septic arthritis after ACL reconstruction. Knee Surg Sports Traumatol Arthrosc. 2014;22(9):2136–44.
180. Warming S, Herzog RB, Lundgaard-Nielsen M, Rathcke MW, Krogsgaard MR. No correlation between performance tests, clinical measurements and data from patient-reported outcome measures (PROM) in children reconstructed for anterior cruciate ligament injury. Knee Surg Sports Traumatol Arthrosc. 2023;31(6):2386–93.
181. Webster KE, Feller JA. The knee adduction moment in hamstring and patellar tendon anterior cruciate ligament reconstructed knees. Knee Surg Sports Traumatol Arthrosc. 2012;20(11):2214–9.
182. Webster KE, Feller JA. Exploring the high reinjury rate in younger patients undergoing anterior cruciate ligament reconstruction. Am J Sports Med. 2016;44.
183. Weiler A, Wagner M, Kittl C. The posterior horn of the lateral meniscus is a reliable novel landmark for femoral tunnel placement in ACL reconstruction. Knee Surg Sports Traumatol Arthrosc 2018;26:1384–1391. https://doi.org/10.1007/s00167-017-4759-4
184. Westermann RW, Wolf BR, Elkins J. Optimizing graft placement in anterior cruciate ligament reconstruction: a finite element analysis. J Knee Surg. 2017;30(02):097–106.
185. Wolf BR, Ramme AJ, Wright RW, Brophy RH, McCarty EC, Vidal AR, et al. Variability in ACL tunnel placement: observational clinical study of surgeon ACL tunnel variability. Am J Sports Med. 2013;41.
186. Xiang X, Chen R, Li R, Gong J, Yang J, Li C, et al. Anterior cruciate ligament reconstruction with femoral direct fiber insertion: a novel technique. Chin Med J (Engl). 2021;135(2):231–3.
187. Xiao Y, Liang Z, Shen S, Liu F, Hu H, Chen B. Increased ACL direct insertion coverage provided more positive biomechanical effects on graft and bone tunnel during knee flexion: a simulation study. J Exp Orthopaed. 2023;10(1):108.
188. Yang H-Y, Cheon J, Choi J, Song E, Seon J. Combined Anterior Cruciate Ligament and Anterolateral Ligament Reconstruction Decreases Passive Anterior Tibial Subluxation Compared With Isolated Anterior Cruciate Ligament Reconstruction Despite Similar Rotational Stability and Clinical Outcomes. Arthrosc J Arthrosc Relat Surg. 2023;39.
189. Yao S, Fu BS, Yung PS. Graft healing after anterior cruciate ligament reconstruction (ACLR). Asia Pac J Sports Med Arthrosc Rehabil Technol. 2021;25:8–15.
190. Yao G, Liu Y, Zhou Z, Zhang X, Liu K, Fu X, et al. A cadaveric study of the optimal isometric region on the anterolateral surface of the knee in anterolateral ligament reconstruction. Orthopaed Surg.
191. Yao S, Yung PSH, Lui PPY. Tackling the challenges of graft healing after anterior cruciate ligament reconstruction—thinking from the endpoint. Front Bioeng Biotechnol. 2021;9.
192. Yoon KH, Kim Y-S, Park J-Y, Kim S-G, Lee J-H, Choi SH, et al. Ideal combination of anatomic tibial and femoral tunnel positions for single-bundle ACL reconstruction. Orthop J Sports Med. 2022;10(1):23259671211069960.
193. Zhang X, Qian Y, Gao F, He C, Guo S, Gao Q, et al. High anteromedial insertion reduced anteroposterior and rotational knee laxity on mid-term follow-up after anatomic anterior cruciate ligament reconstruction. PeerJ. 2023;11:e15898.

194. Zhang Z-Z, Zhang H-Z, Jiang C, Yang R, Chen Z, Song B, et al. Steep posterior tibial slope and excessive anterior tibial translation are associated with increased sagittal meniscal extrusion after posterior lateral meniscus root repair combined with anterior cruciate ligament reconstruction. Arthrosc Sports Med Rehabil. 2024;6:100881.
195. Zheng T, Song G-y, Feng H, Zhang H, Li Y, Li X, et al. Lateral meniscus posterior root lesion influences anterior tibial subluxation of the lateral compartment in extension after anterior cruciate ligament injury. Am J Sports Med. 2020;48(4):838–46.
196. Ziegler CG, Pietrini SD, Westerhaus BD, Anderson CJ, Wijdicks CA, Johansen S. Arthroscopically pertinent landmarks for tunnel positioning in single-bundle and double-bundle anterior cruciate ligament reconstructions. Am J Sports Med. 2011;39.

# Anterolateral Complex (ALC) and Lateral Extra Articular Procedure (LEAP)

## 1 Introduction

Modern ACLR techniques fail to restore native rotational knee kinematics. Even though a central rotatory axis is re-established through ACLR, residual dynamic rotatory laxity, clinically manifested by a positive pivot-shift test, is increasingly recognised as a common finding following ACLR [54]. As residual rotatory laxity is associated with lower PROMS and functional outcomes, the anatomy and biomechanics of the ALC have been revisited and the concept of lateral extra-articular procedures (LEAP) re-introduced as concurrent procedures to ACLR [1, 4, 16, 27, 32, 48, 60, 68, 79]. As tibial cartilage slopes undergo alterations shortly after ACL injury, increased forces on the ACL graft and the ALC based on femoro-tibial kinematics on steeper slopes are observed. The resulting structural changes remain unclear. The anterolateral aspect of the knee represents a conjunction of several distinct, embedded and confluent structures, which synergistically control femoro-tibial kinematics in two functional planes. The exact composition of the ALC is still a matter of scientific debate, partially based on the fact that the direction and sequence of dissection as well as the preservation method of specimen influence the appearance of the ALC and the detectability of its components. The ALC is commonly divided into two major components, the ITB-complex and the capsular complex. The ITB complex comprises the superficial and deep ITB with the Kaplan-fibre mechanism in continuity with the capsulo-osseous layer, which is intimately associated with the joint capsule. The capsular complex comprises a superficial layer and a deep layer. The superficial layer embeds the LCL and corresponds to the ALL, while the deep layer represents the true joint capsule. The confluent conjunction of both layers anterior to the LCL forms a capsular thickening. The concept of a supporting structure within the anterolateral capsule of the knee joint can be found in several early anatomic descriptions. In his desmographic work from 1752 [167], anatomist and founder of syndesmology Josias Weitbrecht described a series of fibres that reinforce the anterolateral joint capsule of the knee, firmly attached to the back of the "*sickle-shaped*



S. Sauer, *ACL Reconstruction: Current Concepts*,
https://doi.org/10.1007/978-3-031-69000-6_4

*cartilage*". In 1872, Friedrich Henle published his observations of anterior fibres of the lateral collateral ligament disappearing into the edge of the lateral meniscus [62]. In 1879, gynaecologist Paul Segond described the eponymous anterolateral tibial avulsion fracture as the result of forced internal tibial rotation and excessive tension of a "*pearly, resistant and fibrous*" band [137]. In contrast to Weitbrecht and Henle, who described the capsular reinforcement as a part of "*the long LCL*" *with* attachments to the anterior fibular neck, Segond's observation implied the existence of a ligamentous structure between the lateral femur and tibia [18]. The concept of a femoro-tibial ligamentous connection was re-introduced by Hughston et al. in the late 1970s. The authors described a 'mid-third lateral capsular ligament' which was observed to be intimately associated with the lateral meniscus, comprising a meniscofemoral and meniscotibial attachment [71]. The structure was thought to be supported superficially by the ITB. In 2012, Vincent et al. published their observations of a consistent lateral structure between the lateral femur and tibial plateau termed the anterolateral ligament [164, 165] which had previously been introduced to describe the capsulo-osseous layer of the ITB (2007). In 2013, Claes et al. published a detailed anatomical description of a new distinct ligamentous structure also termed anterolateral ligament. In contrast to the mid-third-capsular ligament, no association between the ligament and the ITB was observed [18]. The anterolateral ligament described by Claes et al. was found to originate from the lateral epicondyle and not, as observed by Vincent et al., from parts of the popliteus tendon. Even though the existence, entity and biomechanical properties of the ALL as well as the exact constitution of the ALC are still a matter of scientific debate [109, 168], the essential contribution of anterolateral structures of the knee to rotatory knee stability are widely accepted. The detailed description of the ALL and the renewed interest in the ALC has led to a renaissance of lateral extraarticular tenodesis procedures (LET). Current LET's are mostly based on techniques developed by Lemaire and Macintosh. These procedures were strikingly effective in controlling rotatory laxity in the short term, but were abandoned based on recurrent instability, deterioration of subjective scores as well as concerns about over-constraining the lateral compartment with secondary OA development. In contrast to ALL-R, the modified Lemaire tenodesis uses the LCL as a hypomochlion, which is thought to facilitate femoro-tibial reduction towards extension. As biomechanical studies have shown similar kinematic impact of ALL-R and LET, no procedure has emerged to be superior to the other. ALL-R and LET are thought to improve clinical outcomes and reduced failure rates compared to isolated ACLRs in specific indications such as high-grade pivot-shift, RTS to pivoting sports and generalised joint laxity.

## 2 Anatomy of the ALC

The anterolateral aspect of the knee is thought to be constituted of distinct, embedded and confluent structures which synergistically control multi-planar femoro-tibial kinematics. The inherent complexity of the ALC is partially based on the fact the ALC contributes to rotatory control and joint contact while allowing a variable degree of physiological rotatory laxity through range of knee motion. As the anatomic appearance of the ALC has been shown to be influenced by specimen preparation as well as dissection technique, including direction and sequence of exposure, the exact composition of the anterolateral aspect of the knee is still a matter of scientific debate. Different interpretations may also be based on variable focal tension characteristics of the ALC. From a functional perspective, several structures are currently summarised as the anterolateral complex of the knee (ALC) [44, 63, 64]. Current approaches distinguish an ITB complex (comprising the Kaplan-fibre mechanism and the capsulo-osseous layer) from a capsular complex (comprising the ALL/mid-third capsular ligament with menisco-tibial and menisco-femoral attachments).

## 2.1 ITB Complex

The ITB is composed of a superficial, middle, deep and capsulo-osseous layer. The superficial layer of the ITB represent the most prominent structure of the ALC and comprises the iliotibial tract which arises from the aponeurotic coverings of the musculus tensor fascia lata, musculus gluteus maximus, and musculus gluteus medius. Proximally, the superficial ITB is attached to the femur through the lateral intermuscular septum along the linea aspera. In its course, the superficial layer of the ITB runs superficial to the m. vastus lateralis before inserting at the Gerdy tubercle. Anteriorly diverging fibres form the iliopatellar band which inserts at the lateral aspect of the patella and the patellar ligament. Posteriorly diverging fibres reinforce the fascia of the biceps femoris. The middle layer of the ITB comprises the lateral patellofemoral complex and the fascia of the quadriceps femoris, running obliquely from proximal-lateral to distal-medial. The middle layer can only be isolated by sharp dissection. The deep layer of the ITB comprises the Kaplan-fibre mechanism, a tissue condensation of the deep layer which represents the dynamic distal femoral insertion of the superficial ITB. The proximal bundle is characterised by horizontal fibre orientation, inserting distal to the lateral intermuscular septum at the diaphyseal-metaphyseal junction, while the distal bundle displays a longer fibre course inserting at the distal femoral meta-physis which corresponds to the supracondylar flare [52]. The superior lateral genicular artery has been described to be in close proximity to the distal Kaplan-fibre bundle. The tibial insertion site of the deep ITB is located slightly posterior to Gerdy's tubercle in conjunction with the posterior-most fibres of the superficial ITB. A condylar strap arises from the femur and inserts on the deep surface of the ITB. The structure is thought to create a tenodesis effect on the ITB during internal tibial rotation. The retrograde triangular-shaped capsular-osseous layer is thought to be constituted of fibres which originate from the lateral head of the musculus gastrocnemius, musculus plantaris and the posterolateral short head of the musculus biceps femoris. The femoral attachment of the capsulo-osseous layer is found proximally and posteriorly to the lateral femoral epicondyle in continuity with condensations of the deep layer of the ITB. Distally, the capsulo-osseous layer is confluent with the ITB, inserting between the fibular head and Gerdy's tubercle at the lateral tibial tuberosity approximately 5–10 mm below the joint line. In this region, the Segond fracture is typically observed as the result of excessive internal tibial rotation. The capsular-osseous layer tightens excessively in internal tibial rotation and is thought to reinforce the joint capsule, hereby theoretically forming a repositioning loop around the postero-lateral femoral condyle. As the capsulo-osseous layer has more the appearance of a distinct band-like structure rather than a separable tissue layer (Kittl SB), several authors have hypothesised that the capsulo-osseous layer and the ALL may have been mistaken in anatomic dissections.

### 2.2 *Capsular Complex*

The capsular complex corresponds to Seebacher's layer III and can be divided into a superficial and deep lamina dependent on the spatial relationship with the LCL. The superficial lamina embeds the LCL and corresponds to the ALL [6], while the deep lamina lies deep to the the LCL. The confluence of both layers anterior to the LCL forms a capsular thickening which has been associated with the term *mid-third capsular ligament*. The mid-third capsular ligament is not consistently found in contrast to underlying meniscotibial and meniscofemoral attachments. The thin anterior-third capsular ligament represents a layer without significant distinct femoral attachments. The posterior third of the capsule embeds the posterolateral arcuate complex. Even though the ALL has been found to have a cloud like insertional area with significant variations in the literature [84, 85, 100, 139, 152, 153] (similar to the MPFC) the ALL is currently thought to arise proximally and posteriorly to the LCL, running superficially to the LCL and inserting between Gerdy's tubercle and the fibular head approximately 5–10 mm beneath the joint line. The histologic analysis of the ALL supports the entity as a distinct ligament based on the presence of dense, well-arranged connective tissue, mechanoreceptors, terminal nerve endings, as well as a typical ligament-like insertional microarchitecture including a transition to mineralised cartilage [61, 134]. The ALL comprises firm attachments to the lateral meniscus comprising meniscotibial and menisco-femoral attachments [175].

## 3 ALC Biomechanics

The ALC is thought to represent a functional unit of distinct, embedded and confluent structures which synergistically control femoro-tibial kinematics in two functional planes. The superficial plane, represented by the ITB, acts primarily as a ligamentous structure in higher flexion angles [98]. The deep plane, represented by the capsular complex, resists multidirectional forces, and may theoretically be involved in controlling contact forces of the lateral compartment as well as the storage and recovery of elastic energy [8]. The dynamic role of the biceps femoris is not yet fully elucidated but is thought to play a central role in the biomechanics of the ALC. The division of rotatory instability in anteromedial, anterolateral, posteromedial and posterolateral is thought to facilitate the anatomic and biomechanical understanding of rotatory knee instability. However, a growing body of research is emphasising that pathological anterolateral laxity is not necessarily based on insufficiency of anterolateral structures. Vice versa, isolated disruption of anterolateral structures is rarely associated with significantly altered rotational kinematics in the ACL competent knee. ACL deficient knees display increased dynamic rotatory instability, clinically manifested by a positive pivot-shift test, even in the setting of complete ALC integrity. The dominance of stabilising structures is highly dependent on the knee flexion angle. Near extension, the ACL is thought to be the primary restrain against internal tibial rotation, while the ALC becomes more dominant in higher flexion angles. This is reflected in the finding of higher in-situ force in the ACL near knee extension, and higher in-situ force of the ALC in higher flexion angles. In ACL deficiency, the axial rotational axis is thought to be shifted from the tip of the medial tibial intercondylar spine towards the medial border of the knee or beyond [87]. As a result, femoro-tibial rotational kinematics are based on a wider radius which enhances the translatory nature of the motion when an anterior drawer force is applied. As modern ACLR techniques fail to restore native biomechanics, the integrity of the ALC in patients undergoing ACLR is thought to influence the risk of increased residual laxity, risk of subsequent ACLR failure, poor subjective outcomes as well as development of OA. The lateral femoral condyle, in contrast to the medial condyle, undergoes a significant translational movement during knee flexion based on condylar asymmetry and consecutive axial rotation. It has been hypothesised that the lateral femoro-tibial contact area is shifted posteriorly towards the steeper posterior cartilage slope in flexion, increasing the physiological axial rotation laxity envelope. In extension, the femoro-tibial contact area is shifted anteriorly to the relatively flat middle posterior cartilage slope, reducing the axial rotation laxity envelope, hereby minimising the risk of femoro-tibial subluxation in the presence of axial forces. As the anatomy of the ALC is still a matter of scientific debate, there is conflicting evidence regarding the biomechanical properties of its constituting structures. ALC biomechanics are typically assessed by sectioning robotic cadaveric studies [113, 132, 133, 135, 159, 166, 172]. The in vivo validity of the findings is limited as the effects of altered structural synergy, pressure, tension, temperature, damping, friction, DOF, and other factors that affect biomechanical systems, remain unknown. Furthermore, in vivo changes of cartilage slope shortly after ACL injury may alter the significance of the ALC, especially in cases of chronic ACL insufficiency. Findings of systematic reviews are not always comparable based on difference in the applied magnitude of torques and sectioning protocols including management of the ITB. However, basic knowledge regarding the dominance of stabilising structures depending on the knee flexion angle has been derived from robotic studies. Increased internal tibial rotatory laxity is thought to be a central aspect of the pivot-shift test phenomenon. As a result, is has been of clinical interest to identify the structures that represent the primary restraints to tibial internal rotation [2]. Most robotic studies identify the ITB to be the primary restrain to internal tibial rotation. The contribution of the ACL to restraining internal tibial rotation has been shown to be solely significant towards knee extension. The contribution of the capsular complex in restraining internal tibial rotation has been found to be neglectable in most robotic studies. The isolation of the capsular complex may have influenced the results, either by removal of the ITB or by not distinguishing between the ALL and capsular osseous layer sharing the same insertion site. The synergistic working principle of the ALC may pose a challenge in assessing the isolated contribution of a single structure. Forces on isolated structures may represent a causality of a given cutting sequence rather than in vivo in-situ force resistance. Cutting of a last remaining structure in a structural complex will typically induce a significant increase in laxity which does not equate to the in-vivo kinetic behaviour of the structure. The ITB with the Kaplan-fibre mechanism and the capsulo-osseous layer has been found to control internal rotation through a wide range of motion and is thought to contribute to the restrain against femoro-tibial subluxation in the pivot-shift phenomenon [37, 158]. As a result, disruption of the Kaplan-fibre mechanism and the capsulo-osseous layer typically induces increased internal rotation of the tibia throughout a wide range of motion. The role of the capsular complex including the ALL is controversially discussed as biomechanical studies have found variable increase in internal rotatory laxity after sectioning of the ALL and capsular components. Studies in which parts of the inserting ITB were removed, are thought to have overestimated the stabilising effect of the capsular complex. The significance of rotatory laxity in cadaveric studies in higher flexion angles in which the ITB normally reduces the lateral compartment in vivo is unclear. The role of the ALL in the pivot-shift phenomenon is unclear. While Sonnery-Cottet determined the ALL to be involved in controlling internal rotation at 20 and 90 degrees of flexion [147], other authors have failed to identify a significant stabilising contribution of the ALL in lower flexion angles. While several authors have found that the contribution of the ALL to restraining internal tibial rotation is thought to increase significantly with increasing flexion (exceeding the contribution of the ACL in flexion angles beyond 30 degrees [124], other authors have suggested that the ALL acts at the same flexion angles as the ITB in restraining internal tibial rotation and that both structures, together with the lateral capsule, synergistically control internal tibial rotation at higher flexion angles. Other authors have shown a small increase in internal tibial rotation following dissection of the ALL in the ACL deficient knee in extension [150] as well as 30 degrees of flexion (Lording 2015). Dodds et al. found the ALL to be isometric from 0 to 60° of flexion while lengthening with internal tibial rotation, indicating contribution to rotatory control [33]. Depending on the anatomic description and orientation of the ALL, there is conflicting evidence regarding the biomechanical behaviour of the ALL including length changes through range of motion. An ALL arising posteriorly and proximally to the LCL has been found to be relatively isometric, while an ALL arising distally and anteriorly to the LCL has been found to tighten in flexion and loosen in extension, unlikely affecting the pivot-shift test [87]. The ultimate load to failure of the ALL ranges between 50 N and 205 N. The gracilis tendon is currently among the most commonly used grafts for ALL reconstruction. The ultimate load to failure and the young's modulus of the gracilis tendon (200,7 N and 131,7 N/mm respectively) exceed the ultimate load to failure and young's modulus of the ALL (141 N, 21 N/mm, respectively). The biceps femoris and the biceps-capsulo-osseous iliotibial tract confluence are thought to play an important role in rotatory laxity and need to be further investigated.

## 4 Diagnosis of ALC Injury

The diagnosis of ALC injury remains a clinical challenge as the detection of ALC injury by means of imaging modalities and clinical assessment is considered to be limited. Most commonly used image modalities for the diagnosis of ALC injuries include radiography, ultrasound [13] and MRI (Fig. 1). On radiographs, the Segond fracture indicates partial ALC disruption [19, 20]. Radiographic static femoro-tibial subluxation has been associated with high grade pivot-shift, indicative of combined ACL and ALC insufficiency. Similarly, the extend of posterolateral tibial plateau impaction and tibial slope correlate with the incidence of ALC injury. Ultrasound has been found to be useful for the detection of ALC injuries in specific cases, but structure discrimination remains a challenge. The diagnostic accuracy of MRI in regard to ALC integrity is still matter of scientific debate. Even though the detection rate of structures of the ALC on MRI has been reported to be excellent in several studies, the visualisation of an entire structure and differentiation against other adjacent structures is typically compromised. As a result, the reliable detection of ALC injury as well as the assessment of injury complexity by means of MRI is currently regarded to be limited. Indirect findings such as femoro-tibial displacement of the lateral compartment, has been associated with increased MRI based detection of ALC injury [177]. The clinical diagnosis of ALC injury represents a diagnostic challenge. Assessment of ALC integrity is mainly based on the pivot-shift test, which detects dynamic rotatory laxity. The pivot-shift test is positive in the presence of ACL injury even in the setting of complete ALC integrity. A high-grade pivot-shift is thought to be based on concurrent soft-tissue injury, predominantly combined ACL and ALC injuries but is also frequently encountered in meniscal insufficiency. The pivot-shift test is currently not a reliable test in terms of objectiveness and quantitively reliability. Standardisation of the pivot-shift test has been agreed upon in order to improve validity. Navigation systems using dynamic radio-stereometry, stereo-dynamic fluoroscopy, opto-electronic measurement, electromagnetic measurement as well as video-based image analysis are thought to improve the quantitative evaluation of the pivot shift test. Measuring the anterior translation of the lateral tibial plateau rather than global rotation has been proposed to provide a reliable grading of the pivot shift test. According to Zein, the ALL can be visualised through the AL portal with the limb in a figure-of-four-position [176].

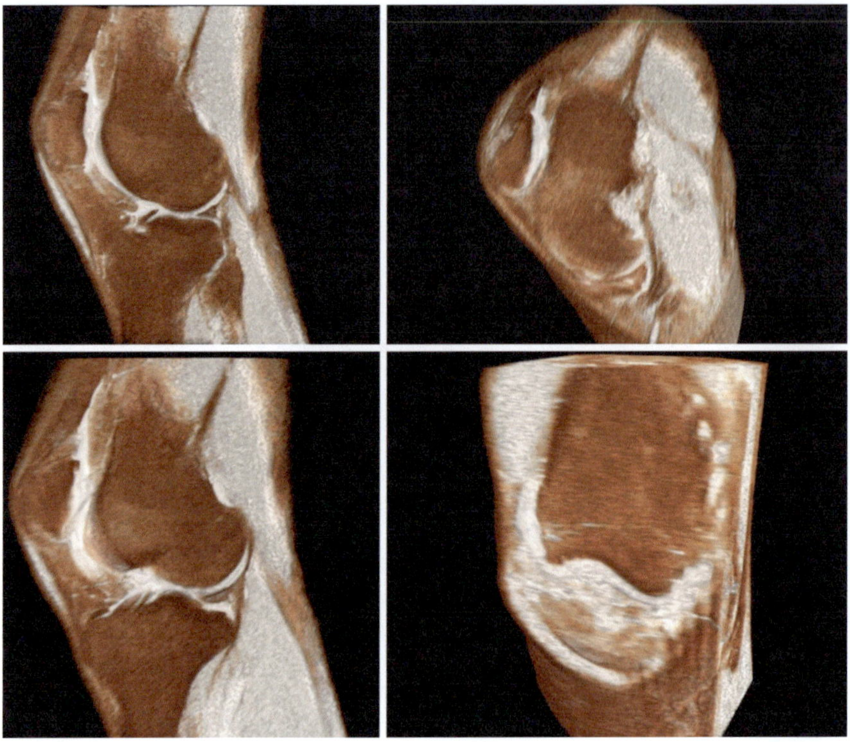

**Fig. 1** 3D MRI may facilitate the assessment of ALC integrity including the Kaplan fibre mechanism

## 5 Lateral Extra Articular Procedures (LEAP)

An emerging body of evidence is indicating that the addition of LEAP to ACLR is associated with improved functional outcomes, reduced residual rotatory laxity and ACLR failure rates [3, 49–51, 68]. As a result, LEAP's have (re)gained substantial scientific attention in recent years [32, 40]. Even though LEAP's have been found to be safe and effective [81], the systematic addition of LEAP to primary and revision ACLR is currently not recommended [138]. LEAP is indicated for patients associated with higher risk of sustaining a recurrent ACL injury, i.e. young patients returning to pivoting sports, displaying a high-grade pivot-shift, increased tibial slope, generalised ligamentous laxity and/or hyperextension. The advantageous effects of LEAP must be weighed against potential risks and complications including increased pain, reduced muscle strength, prolonged recovery time and potential over-constraint of the lateral compartment with consecutive cartilage deterioration [78, 138]. The currently most frequently used LEAP's are the lateral extra-articular tenodesis (LET) and the reconstruction of the anterolateral ligament (ALL-R). Both procedures are typically performed in combination with ACLR but may also be added to a knee with persistent rotatory instability following isolated ACLR. The isolated use of LEAP is reserved to special cases. Anatomic ALL-R is based on the description of the ALL by Claes et al. As the anatomy and function of the ALL are still a matter of scientific debate, several reconstructive techniques have been proposed with variable graft positioning, graft choice, fixation angle as well as recommended graft tension. The current consensus implies that even though the ALL displays a complex cloud like insertional morphology, the femoral insertion area is thought to be located proximal and posterior to the lateral epicondyle (comparable to the MPFC). In ALL-R, a free graft is used which may be incorporated into the ACL graft construct. Current LET procedures are modifications of the Lemaire and Macintosh procedures. The procedures involve a mobilised ITB strip with retained tibial attachment which is typically routed under the LCL and attached to the femur. The main biomechanical difference of LET compared to ALL-R is the more oblique and forceful lever arm of the ITB graft and the pulley-hypomochlion effect of the LCL. As the ITB-graft is tethered by the LCL towards extension, it remains posterior to the axis of rotation and maintains near-isometrical properties. LET and ALL-R demonstrate similar results over isolated ACLR in reducing graft failure rates and controlling residual rotatory laxity [162]. However, as ALL-R represents an anatomic reconstruction and LET a non-anatomical reinforcement, the resulting long-term effects of both procedures need further evaluation.

## 5.1 *Indications of LEAP*

The indications for LEAP in the setting of primary ACLR are currently based on criteria associated with increased risk of ACLR failure. These criteria include age under 25 years with 2 or more of the following factors: returning to pivoting sports, high-grade pivot-shift, joint hyperlaxity (Beighton score exceeding 4), and/or genu recurvatum exceeding 10 degrees [48]. Other relative indications of LEAP include Segond fracture, increased tibial slope, lateral coronal plane laxity, lateral femoral notch sign, reduced MBA, static femoro-tibial displacement, as well as excessive anterior tibial translation following meniscectomy. In addition, LEAP's are typically considered in all revision cases, even though the general benefit is still a matter of scientific debate. Current ACLR techniques do not regenerate the dynamic force transmitting 4-layer anchor architecture of the direct fibres of the ACL. It seems conceivable that the reconstruction of anterolateral structures synergistically supports the ACL-graft, reducing graft strain and facilitating biological healing processes. Especially in chronic cases with increased static femoro-tibial displacement, LEAP is thought to facilitate femoro-tibial reduction towards extension avoiding the femur form articulating with the steep posterior cartilage slope in the presence of axial forces [173]. The presence of lateral compartment OA and posterolateral corner injuries affect the indications of LEAP.

## 5.2 *Anterolateral Ligament Reconstruction (ALL-R)*

### History and Rationale Behind ALL-R

The contribution of the ACL to rotational kinematics is still a matter of scientific debate. However, the pivot-shift test, being almost synonymous to ACL deficiency, is thought to be based on increased tibial rotatory laxity. As residual rotatory laxity is thought to be a significant reason why many athletes do not return to their previous level of sports, normalising native biomechanics has become a central subject of interest in the treatment of ACL injury [53, 84, 147, 148, 159, 177]. As ACL deficiency leads to alteration of cartilage slopes shortly after ACL injury, even anatomically reconstructed ACL grafts may be exposed to increased strain based on kinematics on steeper slopes, and the integrity of the ALL may become more relevant. In ACL deficiency, the axial rotational axis is shifted from the tip of the medial tibial spine towards the medial aspect of the knee or beyond. The resulting rotational movement of the knee is then based on a wider radius and the translational component of the coupled motion is enhanced. As a result, tibial internal rotation is associated with global tibial anterior translation. It is believed that insufficiency of peripheral structures including the ALL may be the underlying cause of variation in rotatory laxity seen in ACL-deficient knees and that repair or reconstruction of the ALL contributes to the normalisation of native knee biomechanics [11, 18, 21, 27, 33, 34, 145, 149]. ALL reconstruction is based on the description of the ALL by Claes et al. [18]. Even though several other authors have been linked to the ALL [21, 71, 137, 164], the detailed description of the ligament by Claes et al. has led to a more systematic approach to reconstructive procedures. The ALL, as part of the ALC, is thought to be involved in the control of rotational knee kinematics [12] and follows the fundamental laws of ligaments. Ligaments undergo elongation based on their kinetic properties as well as external factors including ligament orientation, initial ligament tension and length, joint position, joint geometry, rotatory axes as well as kinematic excursion. The effective function of a ligament is granted within a relatively narrow biomechanical window, exceeding a specific minimal tension to resist loading and remaining under a specific maximal tension prior to plastic deformation and failure. The young's modulus of a ligament determines the amount of elastic energy which is stored during expansion. The purpose of some elastic modules is not necessarily to resist tensile stress but to store and return elastic energy as a biological spring. The ALL is currently thought to display non-isometric properties, tightening in extension to control internal rotation in the presence of axial forces and loosening in flexion to allow for increase of the physiological axial rotatory laxity envelope. As the anatomy and tensile resistance pattern of the ALL are still a matter of scientific debate, ALL-R has been associated with great variability in terms of surgical technique, insertion area, bundle construct, knee angle under graft fixation and ultimately, effect on ACL graft longevity. Since it became evident that ALL grafts need to tighten in extension in order to control rotatory laxity towards knee extension, clinical results of ALL-R have improved. The lateral femoral condyle is thought to have two contact areas.

The switch from the anterior contact area with a wider radius to the posterior contact area with a smaller radius occurs at approximately 15–20 degrees of flexion [77]. Based on different radii, there is no consistent isometric point of the ALL through range of motion. The kinematic influence of the ALL is dependent on ligament orientation including femoral insertion. Variable femoral insertion areas of the ALL are found in the literature. Claes et al. found the femoral insertion to be located slightly anterior to the LCL. Helito et al. found the femoral insertion to be located 2.2 mm anteriorly and 3.5 mm distally to the attachment of the LCL [61]. Dodds et al. found the femoral insertion to be located 8 mm proximally and 4.3 mm posteriorly to the LFE [33]. The tibial insertion of the ALL is typically described to be located halfway between Gerdy's tubercle and the tip of the fibular head, 4.0 mm to 7.0 mm below the joint line. The current consensus is that the femoral insertion of the ALL is located posterior and proximal to the LFE. This position is biomechanically associated with the least length changes of the ALL through range of motion [41]. As the ALL is non-isometric, graft positioning and applied tension under fixation show substantial impact on graft behaviour and joint kinematics. As knee flexion is associated with axial rotation and femoro-tibial displacement, small changes in graft positioning have significant impact on length changes of the ligament. Length changes are influenced by articular geometry and rotatory axes. It is thought to be of importance to secure a graft when the construct reaches its maximum distance between insertional points to avoid joint over-constraint. Recent biomechanical studies emphasise that the ALL plays an important role in restraining internal tibial rotation near knee extension and that ALL injury may aggravate the pivot-shift phenomenon. The reconstruction of the ALL restores native knee biomechanics more closely than isolated ACLR and is currently regarded to be an important aspect of "*physiological ACLR*".

**ALL Reconstruction Procedure**

Several graft options for ALL reconstruction have been described in the literature without one graft emerging as superior to other grafts [14]. ITB grafts come relatively close to the native ALL in terms of young's modulus (39.9 and 21 N/mm respectively), while gracilis tendon grafts significantly exceed the young's modulus of the ALL (131.7 vs. 21 N/mm) [89]. An ALL graft can be incorporated into the ACL construct if the external femoral tunnel aperture of the ACL tunnel is located at the ALL-insertion area. A small incision is made proximal to the LFE. The LFE is identified, and a guide pin is inserted 8 mm proximal and 5–8 mm posterior to the LFE. An incision is made 1 cm below the joint line midway between Gerdy's tubercle and the fibular head. One or two apertures are created on the tibial side. Two apertures (one u-formed tunnel) are thought to better reproduce the broad insertion site of the ALL. Following positioning of the femoral and tibial guide pin, the biomechanical property of the construct is tested with suture tape through complete knee motion. The suture tape should tighten in extension in order to support reposition of the lateral femoro-tibial compartment and loosen in flexion in order to allow for physiological rotatory laxity. The guide pins are then over drilled with a 6 mm reamer. The free graft is inserted into the tunnels and fixed with interference screws or looped through the bone-tunnel. Regardless of surgical technique, the ALL is currently secured in full extension. Graft tension should not exceed 20 N, as internal tibial rotation has been found to be restricted in higher flexion angles when the ALL is over tensioned. Care must be taken to avoid tunnel collision with ACL tunnels. The femoral ACL tunnel should be directed towards the posterior orientation and the femoral ALL tunnel should be aimed at one of the three following orientations: 40° axial and 10° coronal; 35° axial and 5° coronal; or 30° axial and 0° coronal [103].

#### Results of ALL-R

The combination of ALL and ACL reconstruction has been shown to be associated with improved dynamic rotatory laxity as measured with the pivot-shift test and lower graft re-rupture rate when compared to isolated ACL reconstruction [5, 10, 148, 149]. In addition, passive anterior tibial subluxation has been shown to be decreased in combined ACL and ALL reconstruction compared to isolated ACL reconstruction [173]. In terms of subjective scores, there is conflicting evidence on whether combined ACL and ALL reconstruction are superior to isolated ACL reconstruction. While several studies report improved PROM's of combined ALL and ACL reconstruction compared to isolated ACL reconstruction, other studies report comparable subjective scores. De Lima et al. reported improved stability as well as improved Lysholm scores when comparing combined ALL and ACL reconstruction to isolated ACL reconstruction [5]. Sonnery-Cottet et al. reported a significantly lower graft re-rupture rate for combined ALL and ACL reconstruction with 4% compared to isolated ACL reconstruction with 11% (Sonnery-Cottet et al.). In a recent systematic review and meta-analysis, Bosco [10] concluded that combined ALL and ACL reconstruction is associated with improved dynamic residual rotatory laxity, superior PROM's as well as reduced graft failure rates when compared to isolated ACL reconstruction. Furthermore, the addition of ALL-R was found to be non-inferior compared to the addition of LET in combined procedures. Beckers et al. report similar subjective outcome scores when comparing combined ALL and ACL reconstruction to isolated ACL reconstruction (Beckers 2021). Further research is needed to better identify patients who clearly benefit from combined procedures. The potential bias due to lack of patient blinding in randomised controlled trials affecting patient-reported outcomes is well documented and has to be kept in mind [69].

## 5.3 *Lateral Extra Articular Tenodesis (LET)*

#### History and Rationale of LET

First described in detail in 1967 by general surgeon Marcel Lemaire, the eponymous lateral tenodesis is thought to represent one of the foundations of modern

LET procedures. Ultimately, Lemaire intended to improve unsatisfactory results of meniscal surgery, "*palliating ACL deficiency*" by eliminating rotatory laxity [93]. After performing the first isolated tenodesis in 1960 using an ITB strip and a nylon lace, Lemaire published promising results in a series of 46 patients in 1967. Concurrently, Lemaire also suggested that rotatory knee laxity may be associated with a "ressaut *rotatoire*", i.e. a jump within the knee. Lemaire and other authors proposed several tests to assess the phenomenon before Galway and MacIntosh introduced the term *pivot-shift test* at the Canadian Orthopaedic Association meeting in the early nineteen-seventies [42, 43]. The pivot-shift test was thought to assess ACL insufficiency by taking rotatory knee laxity into consideration and a severe pivot-shift phenomenon was thought to be the result of a combined ACL and ALC injury. Following technical descriptions by several authors including Galway, Macintosh and Ellison, LET procedures were popularised. Isolated LET was strikingly effective in controlling rotatory laxity in the short term, but was eventually abandoned based on recurrent laxity, deterioration of subjective outcome scores and concerns regarding long-term consequences of the non-anatomical procedure. Several treatment centres continued with combined ACLR and LET procedures with satisfactory results until an emerging body of evidence challenged the beneficial effect of LET in addition to ACLR and emphasised the importance of a well-performed ACLR over additional procedures and unnecessary sources of morbidity. The current trend supports non-anatomic functional constructions in the sense of a "physiological ACL", rather than an "isolated anatomic ACL". LET is a hypernym for extraarticular procedures involving parts of the ITB to address anterolateral rotatory knee laxity. A strip of the superficial ITB is typically mobilised, retaining its distal insertion at Gerdy's tubercle. The strip is led superficial or deep to the LCL and either attached to the femur through a variety of techniques or folded back and sutured to itself (e.g. ad modum Cocker-Arnold [28]). The deep modified Lemaire tenodesis is currently one of the most commonly used LET procedures. The non-anatomical functional construct is thought to effectively control femoro-tibial kinematics in several planes through a wide range of knee motion [30]. As the ITB strip is routed under the LCL, the graft is kept posterior to the axis of rotation, ensuring near-isometric graft property. The exact position of the proximal femoral attachment is therefore thought to be less influential for near-isometric graft property compared to ALL-R or LET procedures in which the ITB strip is led superficial to the LCL. Tunnel collision with ACL tunnels can be avoided by placing the graft more proximally at the insertion of the distal Kaplan fibres without undesirable biomechanical effects.

### LET (Modified Lemaire Tenodesis)

For the modified (deep) Lemaire tenodesis, the knee is positioned in 80–90 degrees of flexion. A 6–8 cm skin incision is made just posterior to the LFE directed towards Gerdy's tubercle, ending 2 cm prior to it. The subcutaneous tissue is dissected and the superficial layer of the ITB is identified. A strip of 1 cm width and 8–10 cm length is created from the posterior half of the ITB while retaining its insertion at

Gerdy's tubercle. Care must be taken not to damage the underlying LCL. The strip is mobilised and whipstitched with a number 1 Vicryl suture. The underlying LCL is identified (best with the limb in the figure-of-four-position) and small incisions are made anteriorly and posteriorly to the LCL. Care must be taken not to damage the underlying capsule. A tunnel under the LCL is created through blunt dissection and the ITB graft is tunnelled deep to the LCL. The metaphyseal flare is cleared from fat tissue using electrocautery. The insertion, posterior and proximal to the LFE, is identified and a tunnel is created, a suture anchor is placed, or a staple is prepared. The exact position of the femoral attachment does not have significant impact on graft isometry based on the hypomochlion-pulley effect of the LCL. Thus, the graft can be attached more proximally in the area of the distal Kaplan fibres. The LET tunnel can be established under direct visualisation of the ACL tunnel to rule out tunnel violation. The ITB graft is secured with the knee in 60–70 degrees of flexion with the foot in neutral position, holding the graft taut without excessive tension (< 20 N). The open ITB can be adapted but should not be completely closed in order to minimise the risk of over-tensioning the lateral patello-femoral joint [79]. As a salvage procedure or if femoral fixation is unwanted, the graft can be tunnelled under the LCL, folded back and sutured to itself with the knee externally rotated in 30 degrees of flexion (modified Cocker Arnold procedure). The modified Cocker-Arnold procedure has been shown to be non-inferior in terms of clinical outcomes when compared to the modified Lemaire procedure.

## Results of LET

Several clinical studies have investigated the potential advantages of combined ACLR and LET over isolated ACLR. In general, there is sound evidence that LET reduces anterolateral rotatory laxity [79]. As a result, combined procedures are typically associated with improved pivot-shift tests and reduced ACL re-rupture rates when compared to isolated ACLR [48]. However, as even isolated LET may eliminate rotatory laxity, only systematic assessment of ACL integrity by means of MRI (independent of symptomatology) can reveal the exact ACL graft failure rate between groups. Outcome measures including symptomatic instability requiring ACL revision and/or positive or asymmetrical pivot-shift greater than the contralateral side may potentially underreport ACL rupture in specific scenarios. There is conflicting evidence regarding superiority of combined LET and ACLR compared to isolated ACLR in terms of patient related outcomes (Onggo 2022; Park 2023). While several authors report that the combination of ACLR and LET (as well as ALL-R) is associated with significantly improved subjective outcome scores (Aryana 2019; [10]), other authors find lower, similar, or only marginally improved subjective scores of combined ACLR and LET compared to isolated ACLR [48]. The beneficial effect of combined ACLR and LET is thought to be more significant in chronic cases of ACL deficiency (Devitt) in which more pronounced cartilage slope alterations, meniscal deficiency and posterior meniscal extrusion in the sagittal plane are thought to enhance the biomechanical effectiveness of LET in controlling rotatory laxity and reducing ACL graft strain. Even though several studies have reported comparable results in terms of risk of adverse effects and complications of combined ACLR and LET compared to isolated ACLR [48], the systematic addition of LET to primary ACLR is currently not recommended. The potential benefit of combined procedures must be weighted against the risk of potentially increased risk of OA (Castoldi) as well as surgical complications including graft failure, hardware migration, haematoma, infection, chronic pain, muscular hernia, peroneal nerve palsy and knee stiffness (Marshal 2022). As graft re-rupture is typically associated with lower PROM's, the benefit of the LET procedure (reducing graft re-rupture) is thought to outweigh the potential for less severe events such as hardware-irritation or re-operation for its removal (Marmura 2023). In the long term, conversion rate to TKA needs to be considered.

## References


1. Abdelmoneim A, Shannon F. 684 lateral extra-articular tenodesis versus anterolateral ligament reconstruction lateral augmentation for primary anterior cruciate ligament reconstruction with minimum 2-year follow-up: a systematic review and meta-analysis. Br J Surg. 2023;110.
2. Ahsan ZS, Berube EE, Frondorf BJ, Bin Kim H, Marom N, Zayyad ZA, et al. Role of Lateral Extra-articular Tenodesis in Restraining Internal Tibial Rotation: In Vitro Biomechanical Assessment of Lateral Tissue Engagement. The American Journal of Sports Medicine. 2024;52(1):87–7. Albers M, Shaikh H, Herbst E, Onishi K, Nagai K, Musahl V. The iliotibial band and anterolateral capsule have a combined attachment to the Segond fracture. Knee Surg Sports Traumatol Arthrosc. 2018;26.
3. Alessio-Mazzola M, Formica M, Russo A, Sanguineti F, Capello AG, Lovisolo S, et al. Outcome after combined lateral extra-articular tenodesis and anterior cruciate ligament revision in professional soccer players. J Knee Surg. 2018.
4. Andrews JR, Sanders R. A "mini-reconstruction" technique in treating anterolateral rotatory instability (ALRI). Clin Orthop Relat Res. 1983;172:93–96.
5. Ariel de Lima D, de Lima LL, de Souza NGR, de Moraes Perez RA, Sobrado MF, Guimarães TM, Helito CP. Clinical outcomes of combined anterior cruciate ligament and anterolateral ligament reconstruction: a systematic review and meta-analysis. Knee Surg Relat Res. 2021 Sep 23;33(1):33. https://doi.org/10.1186/s43019-021-00115-1. PMID: 34556187; PMCID: PMC8461945.
6. Athanasiou V, Panagopoulos A, Kouzelis A, et al. A Review of Current Concepts of the Anterolateral Complex of the Knee. Orthopedic Reviews. 2022;14(4). https://doi.org/10.52965/001c.38651
7. Bell KM, Rahnemai-Azar AA, Irarrazaval S, Guenther D, Fu FH, Musahl V. In situ force in the anterior cruciate ligament, the lateral collateral ligament, and the anterolateral capsule complex during a simulated pivot shift test. J Orthop Res. 2018;36.
8. Biewener, A. Tendons and Ligaments: Structure, Mechanical Behavior and Biological Function. In: Fratzl, P. (eds) Collagen. Springer, Boston, MA. 2008. https://doi.org/10.1007/978-0-387-73906-9_10
9. Bignozzi S, Zaffagnini S, Lopomo N, Martelli S, Iacono F, Marcacci M. Does a lateral plasty control coupled translation during antero-postérior stress in single-bundle ACL reconstruction? Knee Surg Sports Traumatol Arthrosc. 2009;17.

10. Bosco F, Giustra F, Masoni V, Capella M, Sciannameo V, Camarda L, Massè A, LaPrade RF. Combining an Anterolateral Complex Procedure With Anterior Cruciate Ligament Reconstruction Reduces the Graft Reinjury Rate and Improves Clinical Outcomes: A Systematic Review and Meta-analysis of Randomized Controlled Trials. Am J Sports Med. 2024 Jul;52(8):2129–47. https://doi.org/10.1177/03635465231198494. Epub 2024 Feb 14. PMID: 38353002.
11. Caterine S, Litchfield R, Johnson M, Chronik B, Getgood A. A cadaveric study of the anterolateral ligament: re-introducing the lateral capsular ligament. Knee Surg Sports Traumatol Arthrosc: Off J ESSKA. 2015;23:3186–95. https://doi.org/10.1007/s00167-014-3117-z.
12. Caterine S, Litchfield R, Johnson M, Chronik B, Getgood A. A cadaveric study of the anterolateral ligament: re-introducing the lateral capsular ligament. Knee Surg Sports Traumatol Arthrosc. 2015;23.
13. Cavaignac E, Faruch M, Wytrykowski K, Constant O, Murgier J, Berard E. Ultrasonographic evaluation of anterolateral ligament injuries: correlation with magnetic resonance imaging and pivot-shift testing. Arthroscopy. 2017;33.
14. Chalidis B, Pitsilos C, Kitridis D, Givissis P. Graft choices for anterolateral ligament knee reconstruction surgery: current concepts. World J Clin Cases. 2022;10:8463–73.
15. Chen J, Xu C, Cho E, Huangfu X, Zhao J. Reconstruction for chronic ACL tears with or without anterolateral structure augmentation in patients at high risk for clinical failure: a randomized clinical trial. J Bone Jt Surg Am. 2021;103.
16. Christel P, Djian P. Anterio-lateral extra-articular tenodesis of the knee using a short strip of fascia lata. Rev Chir Orthop Reparatrice Appar Mot. 2002;88.
17. Claes T, Declercq G, Martens M, Lefevre J. Extra-articular ligamentoplasty for chronic ACL insufficiency. Acta Orthop Belg. 1986;52:515–25.
18. Claes S, Vereecke E, Maes M, Victor J, Verdonk P, Bellemans J. Anatomy of the anterolateral ligament of the knee. J Anat. 2013;223:321–8. https://doi.org/10.1111/joa.12087.
19. Claes S, Luyckx T, Vereecke E, Bellemans J. The Segond fracture: a bony injury of the anterolateral ligament of the knee. Arthrosc: J Arthrosc Relat Surg: Off Publ Arthrosc Assoc N Am Int Arthrosc Assoc. 2014;30:1475–1482. https://doi.org/10.1016/j.arthro.2014.05.039
20. Claes S, Luyckx T, Vereecke E, Bellemans J. The Segond fracture: a bony injury of the anterolateral ligament of the knee. Arthroscopy. 2014;30.
21. Claes S, Vereecke E, Maes M, Victor J, Verdonk P, Bellemans J. Anatomy of the anterolateral ligament of the knee. J Anat. 2013;223.
22. Colombet P Jenny JY, Menetrey J, Plaweski S, Zaffagnini S. Current concept in rotational laxity control and evaluation in ACL reconstruction. Orthop Traumatol Surg Res: OTSR. 2012;98:S201–10. https://doi.org/10.1016/j.otsr.2012.10.005
23. Cruells Vieira EL, Vieira EÁ, Teixeira da Silva R, Santos Berlfein PA, Abdalla RJ, Cohen M. An anatomic study of the iliotibial tract. Arthrosc J Arthrosc Relat Surg. 2007;23.
24. Daggett M, Busch K, Sonnery-Cottet B. Surgical dissection of the anterolateral ligament. Arthrosc Tech. 2016;5.
25. Daggett M, Claes S, Helito CP, Imbert P, Monaco E, Lutz C, et al. The role of the anterolateral structures and the ACL in controlling laxity of the intact and ACL-deficient knee: letter to the editor. Am J Sports Med. 2016;44(4):NP14-NP5.
26. Daggett M, Ockuly AC, Cullen M, Busch K, Lutz C, Imbert P, Sonnery-Cottet B. Femoral origin of the anterolateral ligament: an anatomic analysis. Arthrosc: J Arthrosc Relat Surg: Off Publ Arthros Assoc N Am Int Arthrosc Assoc. 2015. https://doi.org/10.1016/j.arthro.2015.10.006
27. DePhillipo NN, Cinque ME, Chahla J, Geeslin AG, LaPrade RF. Anterolateral ligament reconstruction techniques, biomechanics, and clinical outcomes: a systematic review. Arthroscopy. 2017;33.
28. Declercq, Jonas & Schuurmans, Margot & Tack, Lore & Verhelst, Cato & Truijen, Jan. Combined lateral extra-articular tenodesis and anterior cruciate ligament reconstruction: risk of osteoarthritis. European Journal of Orthopaedic Surgery & Traumatology. 2022;33:1–8. https://doi.org/10.1007/s00590-022-03249-4

29. Devitt BM, Bell SE, Ardern CL, Hartwig T, Porter TJ, Feller JA, et al. The role of lateral extra-articular tenodesis in primary anterior cruciate ligament reconstruction: a systematic review with meta-analysis and best-evidence synthesis. Orthop J Sports Med. 2017;5.
30. Devitt BM, Bell SW, Ardern CL, Hartwig T, Porter TJ, Feller JA. The role of lateral extra-articular tenodesis in primary anterior cruciate ligament reconstruction: a systematic review with meta-analysis and best-evidence synthesis. Orthop J Sports Med. 2017;5.
31. Devitt BM, Bouguennec N, Barfod KW, Porter T, Webster KE, Feller JA. Combined anterior cruciate ligament reconstruction and lateral extra-articular tenodesis does not result in an increased rate of osteoarthritis: a systematic review and best evidence synthesis. Knee Surg Sports Traumatol Arthrosc. 2017;25.
32. Dodds AL, Gupte CM, Neyret P, Williams AM, Amis AA. Extra-articular techniques in anterior cruciate ligament reconstruction: a literature review. J Bone Joint Surg Br. 2011;93:1440–1448. https://doi.org/10.1302/0301-620x.93b11.27632
33. Dodds AL, Halewood C, Gupte CM, Williams A, Amis AA. The anterolateral ligament: anatomy, length changes and association with the Segond fracture. Bone Joint J. 2014;96-b:325–331. https://doi.org/10.1302/0301-620x.96b3.33033
34. Dodds AL, Halewood C, Gupte CM, Williams A, Amis AA. The anterolateral ligament: anatomy, length changes and association with the Segond fracture. Bone Jt J. 2014;96-B.
35. Dombrowski ME, Costello JM, Ohashi B, Murawski CD, Rothrauff BB, Arilla FV, Friel NA, Fu FH, Debski RE, Musahl V. Macroscopic anatomical, histological and magnetic resonance imaging correlation of the lateral capsule of the knee. Knee Surg Sports Traumatol Arthrosc. 2015. https://www.legacy.com/us/obituaries/berkshire/name/arthur-ellison-obituary?id=23239614.
36. Ellison AE. Distal iliotibial-band transfer for anterolateral rotatory instability of the knee. J Bone Jt Surg Am. 1979;61.
37. Farinelli L, Meena A, Sonnery-Cottet B, Vieira T, Pioger C, Tapasvi S, et al. Distal Kaplan fibers and anterolateral ligament injuries are associated with greater intra-articular internal tibial rotation in ACL-deficient knees based on magnetic resonance imaging. J Exp Orthop. 2023;10:113.
38. Ferretti A, Gaj E, Andreozzi V, Sonnery-cottet B, Saithna A. Risk factors for grade 3 pivot shift in knees with acute anterior cruciate ligament injuries: a comprehensive evaluation of the importance of osseous and soft tissue parameters from the SANTI study group. Am J Sports Med. 2020;48(10):2408–17.
39. Ferretti A, Monaco E, Fabbri M, Maestri B, De Carli A. Prevalence and classification of injuries of anterolateral complex in acute anterior cruciate ligament tears. Arthrosc J Arthrosc Relat Surg. 2016:1–8. https://doi.org/10.1016/j.arthro.2016.05.010.
40. Ferretti A, Monaco E, Fabbri M, Mazza D, Carli A. The fascia lata anterolateral tenodesis technique. Arthrosc Tech. 2017;6.
41. Forsythe B, Agarwalla A, Lansdown DA, Puzzitiello R, Verma NN, Cole BJ, et al. Proximal fixation anterior to the lateral femoral epicondyle optimizes isometry in anterolateral ligament reconstruction. Knee Surg Sports Traumatol Arthrosc. 2019;27(3):875
42. Galway RD, Beaupre A, MacIntosh DL. Pivot shift: a clinical sign of symptomatic anterior cruciate insufficiency. J Bone Joint Surg (Br). 1972;54:763–4.
43. Galway HR, MacIntosh DL. The lateral pivot shift: a symptom and sign of anterior cruciate ligament insufficiency. Clin Orthop Relat Res. 1980;147:45–50.
44. Garcia-Mansilla I, Zicaro J, Martínez E, Astoul J, Yacuzzi C, Costa-Paz M. Overview of the anterolateral complex of the knee. World J Clin Cases. 2022;10:8474–81.
45. Geeslin AG, Moatshe G, Chahla J, Kruckeberg BM, Muckenhirn KJ, Dornan GJ. Anterolateral knee extra-articular stabilizers: a robotic study comparing anterolateral ligament reconstruction and modified Lemaire lateral extra-articular tenodesis. Am J Sports Med. 2017.
46. Gerdy PN (1829) Anatomie des formes extérieures du corps humain, appliquée à la peinture, à la sculpture et à la chirurgie: Béchet Jeune.
47. Gerdy PN. Chirurgie pratique complète divisée en 7 monographies: Maladies des organes du mouvement, os, muscles, etc., en général: Masson. 1855.

48. Getgood A, Brown C, Lording T, Amis A, Claes S, Geeslin A, et al. The anterolateral complex of the knee: results from the International ALC Consensus Group Meeting. Knee Surg Sports Traumatol Arthrosc. 2019;27(1):166–76.
49. Getgood AMJ, Bryant DM, Litchfield R, Heard M, McCormack RG, Rezansoff A, et al. Lateral extra-articular tenodesis reduces failure of hamstring tendon autograft anterior cruciate ligament reconstruction: 2-year outcomes from the STABILITY study randomized clinical trial. Am J Sports Med. 2020;48(2):285–97.
50. Getgood AMJ, Bryant DM, Litchfield R, Heard M, McCormack RG, Rezansoff A, et al. Lateral extra-articular tenodesis reduces failure of hamstring tendon autograft anterior cruciate ligament reconstruction: 2-year outcomes from the STABILITY Study Randomized Clinical Trial. Am J Sports Med. 2020;48.
51. Getgood A, Bryant D, Firth A, Stability G. The Stability study: a protocol for a multicenter randomized clinical trial comparing anterior cruciate ligament reconstruction with and without lateral extra-articular tenodesis in individuals who are at high risk of graft failure. BMC Musculoskelet Disord. 2019;20.
52. Godin J, Chahla J, Moatshe G, Kruckeberg B, Muckenhirn K, Vap A, et al. A comprehensive reanalysis of the distal iliotibial band: quantitative anatomy, radiographic markers, and biomechanical properties. Am J Sports Med. 2017;45:036354651770796.
53. Goldsmith MT, Turnbull TL, Wijdicks CA, LaPrade RF. The anterolateral ligament: an anatomic, radiographic, and biomechanical analysis. Am J Sports Med. 2015. https://doi.org/10.1177/0363546515578253.
54. Gonzalez-Pola R, Gómez Mont-Landerreche JG, Herrera-Lozano A, Torres-Valdés RA, Flores-Carrillo A. Rotational instability of the knee: Injury of anterior cruciate and anterolateral knee ligaments, MRI findings. J Musculoskelet Surg Res 2021;5:24–9.
55. Guenther D, Griffith C, Lesniak B, Lopomo N, Grassi A, Zaffagnini S. Anterolateral rotatory instability of the knee. Knee Surg Sports Traumatol Arthrosc. 2015;23.
56. Guenther D, Rahnemai-Azar AA, Bell KM, Irarrazaval S, Fu FH, Musahl V. The anterolateral capsule of the knee behaves like a sheet of fibrous tissue. Am J Sports Med. 2017;45.
57. Haims AH, Medvecky MJ, Pavlovich R Jr, Katz LD. MR imaging of the anatomy of and injuries to the lateral and posterolateral aspects of the knee. AJR Am J Roentgenol. 2003;180:647–53.
58. Hamner DL, Brown CH Jr, Steiner ME, Hecker AT, Hayes WC. Hamstring tendon grafts for reconstruction of the anterior cruciate ligament: biomechanical evaluation of the use of multiple strands and tensioning techniques. J Bone Joint Surg Am. 1999;81:549–57.
59. Helito CP, Demange MK, Bonadio MB, Tirico LE, Gobbi RG, Pecora JR, Camanho GL. Anatomy and histology of the knee anterolateral ligament. Orthop J Sports Med. 2013;1:2325967113513546. https://doi.org/10.1177/2325967113513546.
60. Helito CP, Bonadio MB, Gobbi RG, Mota E, Albuquerque RF, Pécora JR, et al. Combined intra- and extra-articular reconstruction of the anterior cruciate ligament: the reconstruction of the knee anterolateral ligament. Arthrosc Tech. 2015;4.
61. Helito CP, Demange MK, Bonadio MB, Tirico LE, Gobbi RG, Pecora JR. Anatomy and histology of the knee anterolateral ligament. Orthop J Sports Med. 2013;1.
62. Henle, J. Handbuch der systematischen Anatomie des Menschen. Vieweg 1873.
63. Herbst E, Albers M, Burnham JM, Fu FH, Musahl V. The anterolateral complex of the knee. Orthop J Sports Med. 2017;5.
64. Herbst E, Albers M, Burnham JM, Shaikh HS, Naendrup JH, Fu FH. The anterolateral complex of the knee: a pictorial essay. Knee Surg Sports Traumatol Arthrosc. 2017;25.
65. Herbst E, Arilla FV, Guenther D, Yacuzzi C, Rahnemai-Azar AA, Fu FH. Lateral extra-articular tenodesis has no effect in knees with isolated anterior cruciate ligament injury. Arthroscopy. 2018;34.
66. Herbst E, Costello J, Popchak A, Tashman S, Irrgang J, Fu F, et al. Untreated injuries to the anterolateral capsular structures do not affect outcomes and kinematics after anatomic anterior cruciate ligament reconstruction. J Clin Med. 2023;12.

67. Hettrich CM, Dunn WR, Reinke EK, Group M, Spindler KP (2013) The rate of subsequent surgery and predictors after anterior cruciate ligament reconstruction: two- and 6-year follow-up results from a multicenter cohort. Am J Sports Med. 41:1534–1540. https://doi.org/10.1177/0363546513490277
68. Hewison CE, Tran MN, Kaniki N, Remtulla A, Bryant D, Getgood AM. Lateral extra-articular tenodesis reduces rotational laxity when combined with anterior cruciate ligament reconstruction: a systematic review of the literature. Arthroscopy. 2015;31.
69. Hróbjartsson A, Emanuelsson F, Skou Thomsen AS, Hilden J, Brorson S. Bias due to lack of patient blinding in clinical trials. A systematic review of trials randomizing patients to blind and nonblind sub-studies. Int J Epidemiol. 2014 Aug;43(4):1272–83. https://doi.org/10.1093/ije/dyu115. Epub 2014 May 30. PMID: 24881045; PMCID: PMC4258786.
70. Hughston JC, Andrews JR, Cross MJ, Moschi A. Classification of knee ligament instabilities. Part I. The medial compartment and cruciate ligaments. J Bone Joint Surg Am. 1976;58:159–72.
71. Hughston JC, Andrews JR, Cross MJ, Moschi A. Classification of knee ligament instabilities. Part II. The lateral compartment. J Bone Joint Surg Am. 1976;58:173–9.
72. Huser LE, Noyes FR, Jurgensmeier D, Levy MS. Anterolateral ligament and iliotibial band control of rotational stability in the anterior cruciate ligament-intact knee: defined by tibiofemoral compartment translations and rotations. Arthroscopy. 2017;33.
73. Inderhaug E, Stephen JM, El-Daou H, Williams A, Amis AA. The effects of anterolateral tenodesis on tibiofemoral contact pressures and kinematics. Am J Sports Med. 2017;45.
74. Inderhaug E, Stephen JM, Williams A, Amis AA. Anterolateral tenodesis or anterolateral ligament complex reconstruction: effect of flexion angle at graft fixation when combined with ACL reconstruction. Am J Sports Med. 2017;45.
75. Inderhaug E, Stephen JM, Williams A, Amis AA. Biomechanical comparison of anterolateral procedures combined with anterior cruciate ligament reconstruction. Am J Sports Med. 2017;45.
76. Ireland J, Trickey EL. Macintosh tenodesis for anterolateral instability of the knee. J Bone Jt Surg Br. 1980;62-B.
77. Iwaki H, Pinskerova V, Freeman MA. Tibiofemoral movement 1: the shapes and relative movements of the femur and tibia in the unloaded cadaver knee. J Bone Joint Surg Br 2000;82:1189–95. https://doi.org/10.1302/0301-620x.82b8.10717
78. Jean-Romain D, Saithna A. Editorial commentary: lateral extra-articular procedures concomitant to anterior cruciate ligament reconstruction must balance clinical efficacy and the risk of kinematic restraint. Arthrosc J Arthrosc Relat Surg. 2022;38:3172–4.
79. Jesani S, Getgood A. Modified Lemaire lateral extra-articular tenodesis augmentation of anterior cruciate ligament reconstruction. JBJS Essent Surg Tech. 2019;9(4):e41.1–7. https://doi.org/10.2106/JBJS.ST.19.00017.
80. Johnson LL. Lateral capsular ligament complex: anatomical and surgical considerations. Am J Sports Med. 1979;7.
81. Kaplan D, Alaia M, Strauss E, Jazrawi L. Anterolateral rotatory instability in the setting of anterior cruciate ligament deficiency. Bull Hosp Joint Dis. 2013;2023(81):24–33.
82. Kaplan EB. The iliotibial tract; clinical and morphological significance. J Bone Joint Surg Am 1958;40-A(4):817–32.
83. Kemkamp WA, Velde SK, Bakker EW, Arkel ER. Anterolateral extra-articular soft tissue reconstruction in anterolateral rotatory instability of the knee. Arthrosc Tech. 2015;4.
84. Kennedy MI, Claes S, Fuso FA, Williams BT, Goldsmith MT, Turnbull TL. The anterolateral ligament: an anatomic, radiographic, and biomechanical analysis. Am J Sports Med. 2015;43.
85. Kennedy MI, Claes S, Fuso FA, Williams BT, Goldsmith MT, Turnbull TL, Wijdicks CA, LaPrade RF. The Anterolateral Ligament: An Anatomic, Radiographic, and Biomechanical Analysis. Am J Sports Med. 2015 Jul;43(7):1606–15. https://doi.org/10.1177/0363546515578253. Epub 2015 Apr 17. PMID: 25888590.
86. Kernkamp WA, Velde SK, Bakker EWP, Arkel ERA. Anterolateral extra-articular soft tissue reconstruction in anterolateral rotatory instability of the knee. Arthrosc Tech. 2015;4.

87. Kittl C, et al.: The role of the anterolateral structures and the ACL in controlling laxity of the intact and ACL-deficient knee. Am J Sports Med. 2015.
88. Kittl C, El-Daou H, Athwal KK, Gupte CM, Weiler A, Williams A. The role of the anterolateral structures and the ACL in controlling laxity of the intact and ACL-deficient knee. Am J Sports Med. 2016;44.
89. Kraeutler MJ, Wolsky RM, Vidal AF, Bravman JT. Anatomy and biomechanics of the native and reconstructed anterior cruciate ligament: surgical implications. J Bone Joint Surg Am 2017;99. https://doi.org/10.2106/JBJS.16.00754
90. LaPrade RF. Arthroscopic evaluation of the lateral compartment of knees with grade 3 posterolateral knee complex injuries. Am J Sports Med. 1997;25:596–602.
91. Lane CG, Warren R, Pearle AD. The pivot shift. J Am Acad Orthop Surg. 2008;16:679–88.
92. Lee JK, Seo YJ, Jeong S-Y, Yang J-H. Biomechanical function of the anterolateral ligament of the knee: a systematic review. Knee Surg Relat Res. 2020;32(1):6.
93. Lemaire, M. "Rupture anciennes du ligament croisé antérieur. Frequence-clinique traitement." J Bone Jt Surg Br B 1967;58:142.
94. Lerat JL, Moyen B, Garin C, Mandrino A, Besse JL, Brunet-Guedj E. Anterior laxity and internal arthritis of the knee. Results of the reconstruction of the anterior cruciate ligament associated with tibial osteotomy. Rev Chir Orthop Reparatrice Appar Mot. 1993;79.
95. Lording T, Corbo G, Bryant D, Burkhart TA, Getgood A. Rotational laxity control by the anterolateral ligament and the lateral meniscus is dependent on knee flexion angle: a cadaveric biomechanical study. Clin Orthop Relat Res. 2017:475.
96. Louis ML, D'ingrado P, Ehkirch FP, Bertiaux S, Colombet P, Sonnery-Cottet B, et al. Combined intra- and extra-articular grafting for revision ACL reconstruction: a multicentre study by the French Arthroscopy Society (SFA). Orthop Traumatol Surg Res. 2017;103.
97. Lubowitz JH, Provencher MT, Brand JC, Rossi MJ. The knee anterolateral ligament. Arthroscopy. 2014;30.
98. Lutz C, Sonnery-Cottet B, Niglis L, Freychet B, Clavert P, Imbert P. Behavior of the anterolateral structures of the knee during internal rotation. Orthop Traumatol Surg Res: OTSR. 2015;101:523–8. https://doi.org/10.1016/j.otsr.2015.04.007.
99. MacIntosh D. Lateral substitution reconstruction. J Bone Jt Surg. 1976;58:142.
100. Macchi V, Porzionato A, Morra A, Stecco C, Tortorella C, Menegolo M, Grignon B, De Caro R. The anterolateral ligament of the knee: a radiologic and histotopographic study. Surg Radiol Anat: SRA. 2015. https://doi.org/10.1007/s00276-015-1566-9
101. Meredick RB, Vance KJ, Appleby D, Lubowitz JH. Outcome of single-bundle versus double-bundle reconstruction of the anterior cruciate ligament: a meta-analysis. Am J Sports Med. 2008;36:1414–21. https://doi.org/10.1177/0363546508317964.
102. Miller TK. The role of an extra-articular tenodesis in revision of anterior cruciate ligament reconstruction. Clin Sports Med. 2018;37.
103. Mitrousias V, Chalatsis G, Komnos G, Neri T, Hantes M. Lateral augmentation procedures in anatomic anterior cruciate ligament reconstruction. How to avoid tunnel collision with intraoperative tunnel visualization: A technical note. J ISAKOS. 2023 Jun;8(3):137–9. https://doi.org/10.1016/j.jisako.2023.03.001. Epub 2023 Mar 13. PMID: 36921765.
104. Mogos Ş, Antonescu D, Stoica I-C, D'Ambrosi R. Superior rotational stability and lower re-ruptures rate after combined anterolateral and anterior cruciate ligament reconstruction compared to isolated anterior cruciate ligament reconstruction: a 2-year prospective randomized clinical trial. Phys Sportsmed. 2023;51(4):371–8.
105. Monaco E, Ferretti A, Labianca L, Maestri B, Speranza A, Kelly MJ, D'Arrigo C. Navigated knee kinematics after cutting of the ACL and its secondary restraint. Knee Surg Sports Traumatol Arthrosc: Off J ESSKA. 2012;20:870–7. https://doi.org/10.1007/s00167-011-1640-8.
106. Moorman CT 3rd, LaPrade RF. Anatomy and biomechanics of the posterolateral corner of the knee. J Knee Surg. 2005;18:137–45.
107. Morgan AM, Bi AS, Kaplan DJ, Alaia MJ, Strauss EJ, Jazrawi LM. An eponymous history of the anterolateral ligament complex of the knee. Knee Surg Relat Res. 2022;34(1):45.

108. Murgier J, Devitt BM, Sevre J, Feller JA, Cavaignac E. The origin of the knee anterolateral ligament discovery: a translation of Segond's original work with commentary. Arthrosc J Arthrosc Relat Surg. 2019;35.
109. Musahl V, Rahnemai-Azar AA, van Eck CF, Guenther D, Fu FH. Anterolateral ligament of the knee, fact or fiction? Knee Surg Sports Traumatol Arthrosc. 2016;24(1):2–3.
110. Musahl V. Rotatory knee laxity and the pivot shift. Knee Surg Sports Traumatol Arthrosc. 2012;20.
111. Musahl V, Burnham J, Lian J, Popchak A, Svantesson E, Kuroda R, et al. High-grade rotatory knee laxity may be predictable in ACL injuries. Knee Surg Sports Traumatol Arthrosc. 2018.
112. Nazzal E, Keeling L, Ryan P, Herman Z, Hughes J. The role of lateral extra-articular tenodesis in anterior cruciate ligament reconstruction and treatment of rotatory knee instability: a scoping review. Curr Rev Musculoskelet Med. 2023;16:1–11.
113. Nitri M, Rasmussen MT, Williams BT, Moulton SG, Cruz RS, Dornan GJ, Goldsmith MT, LaPrade RF. An in vitro robotic assessment of the anterolateral ligament, Part 2: anterolateral ligament reconstruction combined with anterior cruciate ligament reconstruction. Am J Sports Med. 2016;44:593–601. https://doi.org/10.1177/0363546515620183.
114. Norwood LA Jr, Andrews JR, Meisterling RC, Glancy GL. Acute anterolateral rotatory instability of the knee. J Bone Joint Surg Am. 1979;61:704–9.
115. Norwood LA, Andrews JR, Meisterling RC, Glancy GL. Acute anterolateral rotatory instability of the knee. J Bone Joint Surg Am. 1979;61.
116. Noyes FR, Barber SD. The effect of an extra-articular procedure on allograft reconstructions for chronic ruptures of the anterior cruciate ligament. J Bone Joint Surg Am. 1991;73.
117. Noyes FR, Grood ES, Cummings JF, Wroble RR. An analysis of the pivot shift phenomenon. The knee motions and subluxations induced by different examiners. Am J Sports Med. 1991;19.
118. Noyes FR, Huser LE, Jurgensmeier D, Walsh J, Levy MS. Is an anterolateral ligament reconstruction required in ACL-reconstructed knees with associated injury to the anterolateral structures? Am J Sports Med. 2017;45.
119. Noyes FR, Huser LE, Jurgensmeier D, Walsh J, Levy MS. Is an anterolateral ligament reconstruction required in ACL-reconstructed knees with associated injury to the anterolateral structures? A robotic analysis of rotational knee stability. Am J Sports Med. 2017;45.
120. Noyes FR, Huser LE, Levy MS. Rotational knee instability in ACL-deficient knees: role of the anterolateral ligament and iliotibial band as defined by tibiofemoral compartment translations and rotations. J Bone Jt Surg Am. 2017;99.
121. Noyes FR, Huser LE, Levy MS. Rotational knee instability in ACL-deficient knees: role of the anterolateral ligament and iliotibial band as defined by tibiofemoral compartment translations and rotations. J Bone Joint Surg Am. 2017;99.
122. Ntagiopoulos P, Dejour D. Extra-articular plasty for revision anterior cruciate ligament reconstruction. Clin Sports Med. 2018;37.
123. O'Brien SJ, Warren RF, Wickiewicz TL, Rawlins BA, Allen AA, Panariello R. The iliotibial band lateral sling procedure and its effect on the results of anterior cruciate ligament reconstruction. Am J Sports Med. 1991;19.
124. Parsons EM, Gee AO, Spiekerman C, Cavanagh PR. The biomechanical function of the anterolateral ligament of the knee. Am J Sports Med. 2015;43:669–74. https://doi.org/10.1177/0363546514562751.
125. Parsons EM, Gee AO, Spiekerman C, Cavanagh PR. The biomechanical function of the anterolateral ligament of the knee. Am J Sports Med. 2015;43.
126. Pavão DM, Cruz RS, Faria JLR, Sousa EB, Barretto JM. Modified Lemaire lateral tenodesis associated with an intra-articular reconstruction technique with bone-tendon-bone graft using an adjustable fixation mechanism. Arthrosc Tech. 2019;8.
127. Pearl AJ, Bergfeld JA (1992) Extra-articular reconstruction in the anterior cruciate ligament deficient knee. Am Orthop Soc Sports Med.
128. Peltier A, Lording T, Maubisson L, Ballis R, Neyret P, Lustig S. The role of the meniscotibial ligament in posteromedial rotational knee stability. Knee Surg Sports Traumatol Arthrosc 2015;23. https://doi.org/10.1007/s00167-015-3751-0

129. Perelli S, Costa GG, Montiel V, Formagnana M, Bait C, Espregueira-Mendes J, et al. Combined anterior cruciate ligament reconstruction and modified lemaire lateral extra-articular tenodesis better restores knee stability and reduces failure rates than isolated anterior cruciate ligament reconstruction in skeletally immature patients. Am J Sports Med. 2022;50:3635465221128926.
130. Puddu G, Ferretti A, Mariani PP, Conteduca F. Le lesioni isolate del legamento crociato anteriore. Il Ginocchio. 1987.
131. Rahnemai-Azar AA, Miller RM, Guenther D, Fu FF, Lesniak B, Musahl V, Debski RE. Structural Properties of the Anterolateral Capsule and Iliotibial Band of the Knee. Podium Presented in Summer Biomechanics, Bioengineering, and Biotransport Conference in June 2015 Utah and in American Academy of Orthopaedic Surgeons meeting; Orlando, FL. 2016.
132. Rasmussen MT, Nitri M, Williams BT, Moulton SG, Cruz RS, Dornan GJ, Goldsmith MT, LaPrade RF. An in vitro robotic assessment of the antero-lateral ligament, Part 1: secondary role of the anterolateral ligament in the setting of an anterior cruciate ligament injury. Am J Sports Med. 2015. https://doi.org/10.1177/0363546515618387.
133. Rasmussen MT, Nitri M, Williams BT, Moulton SG, Cruz RS, Dornan GJ, Goldsmith MT, LaPrade RF. An in vitro robotic assessment of the anterolateral ligament, Part 1: secondary role of the anterolateral ligament in the setting of an anterior cruciate ligament injury. Am J Sports Med. 2016;44(3):585–92.
134. Sabatini L, Capella M, Vezza D, Barberis L, Camazzola D, Risitano S, Drocco L, Massè A. Anterolateral complex of the knee: State of the art. World J Orthop. 2022 Aug 18;13(8):679–92. https://doi.org/10.5312/wjo.v13.i8.679. PMID: 36159618; PMCID: PMC9453282.
135. Saiegh YA, Suero EM, Guenther D, Hawi N, Decker S, Krettek C. Sectioning the anterolateral ligament did not increase tibiofemoral translation or rotation in an ACL-deficient cadaveric model. Knee Surg Sports Traumatol Arthrosc. 2017;25.
136. Salmon L, Russell V, Musgrove T, Pinczewski L, Refshauge K. Incidence and risk factors for graft rupture and contralateral rupture after anterior cruciate ligament reconstruction. Arthrosc: J Arthrosc Relat Surg: Off Publ Arthrosc Assoc N Am Int Arthrosc Assoc. 2005;21:948–957. https://doi.org/10.1016/j.arthro.2005.04.110. Segond P. Recherches cliniques et expérimentales sur les épanchements sanguins du genou par entorse. Paris: Progrès Médical; 1879. Accessible from http://www.patrimoineedilivre.com/. p 1–85.
137. Segond P. Recherches cliniques et experimentales sur les epanchements sanguins du genou par entorse. Progres Medical. 1879. http://www.patrimoine.edilivre.com.
138. Servant C. Editorial Commentary: During Anterior Cruciate Ligament Reconstruction, Lateral Extra-Articular Procedures Have Risks and Should be Reserved for Proper Indications: Do Not LET ALL Revision Anterior Cruciate Ligament Reconstructions Be the Same. Arthroscopy 2023;39:320–3. https://doi.org/10.1016/j.arthro.2022.08.028.
139. Shea KG, Milewski MD, Cannamela PC, Ganley TJ, Fabricant PD, Terhune EB, et al. Anterolateral ligament of the knee shows variable anatomy in pediatric specimens. Clin Orthop Relat Res. 2016;475.
140. Smeets K, Slane J, Scheys L, Forsyth R, Claes S, Bellemans J. The anterolateral ligament has similar biomechanical and histologic properties to the inferior glenohumeral ligament. Arthroscopy. 2017;33.
141. Smith JO, Yasen SK, Lord B, Wilson AJ. Combined anterolateral ligament and anatomic anterior cruciate ligament reconstruction of the knee. Knee Surg Sports Traumatol Arthrosc: Off J ESSKA. 2015;23:3151–6. https://doi.org/10.1007/s00167-015-3783-5.
142. Song GY, Zhang H, Zhang J, Liu X, Xue Z, Qian Y, et al. Greater static anterior tibial subluxation of the lateral compartment after an acute anterior cruciate ligament injury is associated with an increased posterior tibial slope. Am J Sports Med. 2018;46(7):1617–23.
143. Song GY, et al.: Risk Factors Associated With Grade 3 Pivot Shift After Acute Anterior Cruciate Ligament Injuries. Am J Sports Med. 2015.
144. Sonnery-Cottet B, Lutz C, Daggett M, Dalmay F, Freychet B, Niglis L, Imbert P. The involvement of the anterolateral ligament in rotational control of the knee. Am J Sports Med. 2016. https://doi.org/10.1177/0363546515625282.

145. Sonnery-Cottet B, Thaunat M, Freychet B, Pupim BH, Murphy CG, Claes S. Outcome of a combined anterior cruciate ligament and anterolateral ligament reconstruction technique with a minimum 2-year followup. Am J Sports Med. 2015. https://doi.org/10.1177/0363546515571571.
146. Sonnery-Cottet B, Barbosa N, Tuteja S, Daggett D, Kajetanek C, Thaunat M. Minimally invasive anterolateral ligament reconstruction in the setting of ACL injury. Arthrosc Tech 2016;5(1):e211–5. https://doi.org/10.1016/j.eats.2015.11.005
147. Sonnery-Cottet B, Claes S, Blakeney WG, Cavaignac E, Saithna A, Daggett M, et al. Anterolateral ligament: let's stick to the facts! Arthrosc J Arthrosc Relat Surg. 2018;34.
148. Sonnery-Cottet B, Saithna A, Cavalier M, Kajetanek C, Temponi EF, Daggett M. Anterolateral ligament reconstruction is associated with significantly reduced ACL graft rupture rates at a minimum follow-up of 2years: a prospective comparative study of 502 patients from the SANTI study group. Am J Sports Med. 2017;45.
149. Sonnery-Cottet B, Thaunat M, Freychet B, Pupim BH, Murphy CG, Claes S. Outcome of a combined anterior cruciate ligament and anterolateral ligament reconstruction technique with a minimum 2-year follow-up. Am J Sports Med. 2015;43.
150. Spencer L, Burkhart TA, Tran MN, Rezansoff AJ, Deo S, Caterine S, Getgood AM. Biomechanical analysis of simulated clinical testing and reconstruction of the anterolateral ligament of the knee. Am J Sports Med. 2015;43:2189–97. https://doi.org/10.1177/0363546515589166.
151. Stensbirk F, Thorborg K, Konradsen L, Jørgensen U, Hölmich P. Iliotibial band autograft versus bone-patella-tendon-bone autograft, a possible alternative for ACL reconstruction: a 15-year prospective randomized controlled trial. Knee Surg Sports Traumatol Arthrosc. 2014;22.
152. Stijak L, Bumbasirevic M, Radonjic V, Kadija M, Puskas L, Milovanovic D, Filipovic B. Anatomic description of the anterolateral ligament of the knee. Knee Surg Sports Traumatol Arthrosc: Off J ESSKA; 2014. https://doi.org/10.1007/s00167-014-3422-6
153. Stijak L, Bumbasirevic M, Radonjic V, Kadija M, Puskas L, Milovanovic D, Filipovic B. Anatomic description of the anterolateral ligament of the knee. Knee Surg Sports Traumatol Arthrosc. 2014.
154. Strickland J, Fester E, Noyes FR. Lateral and posterior knee anatomy. Noyes' knee disorders: surgery, rehabilitation, clinical outcomes. Philadelphia: Elsevier; 2017.
155. Sudasna S, Harnsiriwattanagit K. The ligamentous structures of the posterolateral aspect of the knee. Bull Hosp Joint Dis Orthop Inst. 1990;50.
156. Suero EM, Njoku IU, Voigt MR, Lin J, Koenig D, Pearle AD. The role of the iliotibial band during the pivot shift test. Knee Surg, Sports Traumatol, Arthrosc: Off J ESSKA. 2013;21.
157. Suomalainen P, Jarvela T, Paakkala A, Kannus P, Jarvinen M. Double-bundle versus single-bundle anterior cruciate ligament reconstruction: a prospective randomized study with 5-year results. Am J Sports Med. 2012;40:1511–8. https://doi.org/10.1177/036354651244817746.
158. Tanaka M, Vyas D, Moloney G, Bedi A, Pearle AD, Musahl V. What does it take to have a high-grade pivot shift? Knee Surg Sports Traumatol Arthrosc: Off J ESSKA. 2012;20:737–42. https://doi.org/10.1007/s00167-011-1866-5.
159. Tavlo M, Eljaja S, Jensen JT, Siersma VD, Krogsgaard MR. The role of the anterolateral ligament in ACL insufficient and reconstructed knees on rotatory stability: a biomechanical study on human cadavers. Scand J Med Sci Sports. 2015. https://doi.org/10.1111/sms.12524.
160. Terry GC, Hughston JC, Norwood LA. The anatomy of the iliopatellar band and iliotibial tract. Am J Sports Med. 1986;14:39–45.
161. Tjong VK, Whelan DB. The MacIntosh procedure. Rotatory knee instability: an evidence based approach. Cham: Springer International Publishing; 2017.
162. van der Wal WA, Meijer DT, Hoogeslag RAG, LaPrade RF. The Iliotibial Band is the Main Secondary Stabilizer for Anterolateral Rotatory Instability and both a Lemaire Tenodesis and anterolateral ligament reconstruction can restore native knee kinematics in the ACL reconstructed knee. A systematic review of biomechanical cadaveric studies. Arthroscopy. 2023.

163. Vieira EL, Vieira EA, da Silva RT, Berlfein PA, Abdalla RJ, Cohen M. An anatomic study of the iliotibial tract. Arthrosc: J Arthrosc Relat Surg: Off Publ Arthrosc Assoc N Am Int Arthrosc Assoc. 2007;23:269–274. https://doi.org/10.1016/j.arthro.2006.11.019, S0749–8063(06)01443–5 (pii)
164. Vincent JP, Magnussen RA, Gezmez F, Uguen A, Jacobi M, Weppe F, Al-Saati MF, Lustig S, Demey G, Servien E, Neyret P. The anterolateral ligament of the human knee: an anatomic and histologic study. Knee Surg Sports Traumatol Arthrosc: Off J ESSKA. 2012;20:147–252. https://doi.org/10.1007/s00167-011-1580-3.
165. Vincent JP, Magnussen RA, Gezmez F, Uguen A, Jacobi M, Weppe F, et al. The anterolateral ligament of the human knee: an anatomic and histologic study. Knee Surg Sports Traumatol Arthrosc. 2012;20.
166. Wal W, Meijer D, Hoogeslag R, LaPrade R. The iliotibial band is the main secondary stabilizer for anterolateral rotatory instability and both a Lemaire tenodesis and anterolateral ligament reconstruction can restore native knee kinematics in the ACL reconstructed knee. Systematic review of biomechanical cadaveric studies. Arthrosc J Arthrosc Relat Surg. 2023.
167. Weitbrecht, J. Desmographie ou description des ligamens du corps humain, avec figures. chez Durand 1752.
168. Williams A. Editorial commentary: the anterolateral ligament: the emperor's new clothes? Arthrosc J Arthrosc Relat Surg. 2018;34.
169. Willinger L, Athwal K, Holthof S, Imhoff A, Williams A, Amis A. Role of the anterior cruciate ligament, anterolateral complex, and lateral meniscus posterior root in anterolateral rotatory knee instability: a biomechanical study. Am J Sports Med. 2023;51:036354652311610.
170. Wright RW, Magnussen RA, Dunn WR, Spindler KP. Ipsilateral graft and contralateral ACL rupture at five years or more following ACL reconstruction: a systematic review. J Bone Joint Surg Am. 2011;93:1159–65. https://doi.org/10.2106/JBJS.J.00898.
171. Wroble RR, Grood ES, Cummings JS, Henderson JM, Noyes FR. The role of the lateral extraarticular restraints in the anterior cruciate ligament-deficient knee. Am J Sports Med 1993;21:257–262; discussion 263.
172. Yamamoto Y, Hsu WH, Fisk JA, Scyoc AH, Miura K, Woo SL. Effect of the iliotibial band on knee biomechanics during a simulated pivot shift test. J Orthop Res: Off Publ Orthop Res Soc. 2006;24.
173. Yang, S., Liu, Y., Ma, S., Ding, C., Kong, Z., Li, H., Huang, F., Chen, H. & Zhong, H.. 2023. Stress and strain changes of the anterior cruciate ligament at different knee flexion angles: A three-dimensional finite element study. J Orthop Sci https://doi.org/10.1016/j.jos.2023.05.015
174. Yao G, Liu Y, Zhou Z, Zhang X, Liu K, Fu X, et al. A cadaveric study of the optimal isometric region on the anterolateral surface of the knee in anterolateral ligament reconstruction. Orthopaed Surg.
175. Zaffagnini S, Grassi A, Marcheggiani Muccioli GM, Raggi F, Romagnoli M, Bondi A, et al. The anterolateral ligament does exist: an anatomic description. Clin Sports Med. 2018;37.
176. Zein AM. Step-by-Step Arthroscopic Assessment of the Anterolateral Ligament of the Knee Using Anatomic Landmarks. Arthrosc Tech. 2015 Dec 14;4(6):e825–31. https://doi.org/10.1016/j.eats.2015.08.002. PMID: 27284519; PMCID: PMC4886523.
177. Zheng T, Song G, Wang C, Li Y, Zhang Z, Cao Y, et al. Effect of anterolateral ligament status and inherent knee anatomy on anterior tibial subluxation of the lateral compartment after acute anterior cruciate ligament injury: a cohort study based on MRI analysis. Am J Sports Med. 2023;51(4):968–76.

# Paediatric ACL Injuries

## 1 Introduction

Over the past decades, a global and concerning increase of paediatric ACL injuries has been observed [20, 32, 63, 120]. Even though an intensified focus on paediatric ACL injuries has increased detection rates, professional demands being placed on young athletes have undoubtedly increased the susceptibility to paediatric ACL injuries [30]. ACL related injuries account for approximately one-third of paediatric knee injuries in football players between the ages of 5 and 18 years and comprise cartilaginous and bony ACL avulsions as well as partial and complete ACL tears [113]. In general, the ACL injury pattern is thought to correspond to the general injury pattern of children with decreased injury risk during the ages 6–12 years and increasing injury risk with advancing age and trauma exposition [111]. ACL injury risk begins to increase significantly at 12–13 years of age in girls, and at 14–15 years of age in boys [67]. In the treatment of paediatric ACL related injuries, recurrent instability with consecutive chondral and meniscal injury associated with non-operative treatment [53, 119] must be weighed against surgical complications including growth disturbance. Delayed operative treatment is regarded as an option with the advantage of physical and psychological maturation of the patient [123]. However, based on the potential risk of irreparable meniscus and/or cartilage injury associated with non-operative treatment [53], the current trend supports early ACLR for the treatment of the unstable ACL deficient knee [36, 41]. High level evidence on optimal treatment of paediatric ACL deficiency is scarce. Even though the incidence of growth plate disturbance as a complication of ACLR is thought to be underreported, it is currently thought to be comparable to the risk of septic arthritis following ACLR (Wong) [121]. ACL injury is associated with a significant impact on quality of life of young patients. Even after successful ACLR, graft rupture or contralateral ACL injury as well as further surgical interventions are common. The discontinuation of sports-related social contact may play a crucial psychological role. In recent years, the paediatric population has received increased scientific attention



S. Sauer, *ACL Reconstruction: Current Concepts*,
https://doi.org/10.1007/978-3-031-69000-6_5

with emphasis on specific characteristics of the paediatric ACL such as size, kinetic properties including young's modulus, fibre maturity and spatial course in order to optimise treatment approaches of ACL injuries. Furthermore, focus on the female athlete, displaying higher quadriceps-hamstring activation ratio [1] and higher risk of ACL injury per athletic exposure, is steadily increasing [45, 67]. Anatomic factors including increased tibial slope and less well-defined ALL, as well as growth related factors with surgical implications are being considered. While the distance of the physis to the femoral insertion area of the ACL is thought to remain relatively consistent during growth, the distance of the proximal tibial physis to the tibial insertion area of the ACL changes during growth. The intercondylar notch undergoes significant growth and widening until the age of 11 years and the ACL changes angulation with increasing age becoming more vertical until the age of 18 years. The lateral intercondylar ridge becomes more distinct, and several structures of the knee display increasing young's modulus with advancing age. Inflammatory responses in younger knees have been shown to more effectively support healing processes. On the other hand, the paediatric population shows typically lower compliance to rehabilitation protocols and the restoration of neuromuscular activity and muscle mass is typically delayed compared to adults. Several paediatric ACLR techniques including physeal sparing and transphyseal techniques have been described in the literature associated with promising results, albeit data on long term outcomes and complication rates are typically scarce. All surgical techniques are associated with relatively high graft re-rupture rates [98]. Prevention programs are thought to be of paramount importance. However, the implementation of these programs represents a challenge.

## 2 Trauma Mechanism

Paediatric ACL injuries are predominantly the result of non-contact deceleration or landing manoeuvres, pivoting motions or hyper-extensional knee excursions [15, 30]. ACL-injury-provoking joint positions comprising hip flexion, slight knee flexion and a planted foot, especially on high friction surfaces (Taylor 2012; Drakos 2013) have been shown to significantly increase the risk of ACL injury (Carlson 2016). The exact ACL compromising trauma is often not elicitable, or the more noticeable knee collapse is reported. Newest research suggests that non-contact ACL injury may be predominantly the result of axial forces while rotational torque and valgus loading may represent contributing factors associated with ACL injury. There is a growing body of research highlighting the substantial but overlooked impact of external rotation on ACL stress and injury risk (Santos 2023). It has been hypothesised that the femorotibial subluxation driven by axial forces is unlikely to be avoided by reflexive muscle stabilisation as the peak ground reaction force is thought to induce femorotibial subluxation in under 40 ms, while reflexive muscle stabilisation is typically established after 100 ms (Hewett 2011). The influence of quadriceps-contraction on axial forces has been elucidated but remains unclear. The degree of tibial tubercle ossification and resulting impact on ACL injury risk is currently elucidated. Geometrical factors including increased anterior pelvic tilt, increased femoral anteversion, decreased intercondylar notch width, decreased MBA as well as increased posterior tibial slope have been shown to potentially modulate ACL injury risk [1, 97, 111] (Dare 2015; Swami 2013; Christensen 2015; Vyas 2011). Different radii of contact areas of the lateral femoral condyle are thought to be associated with increased risk of ACL injury. From approximately 0–20 degrees of flexion, the lateral femoral condyle articulates through the anterior femoral contact area. The relatively short anterior contact area has a larger radius than the posterior contact area. Joint contact on the flat, anterior contact area of the lateral femoral condyle favours sliding over rolling in the presence of axial compressive forces [16]. As cartilage slopes may undergo steepening shortly after ACL injury, even an anatomic ACL graft can potentially be exposed to increased strain based on kinematics on steeper slopes (Sauer ISAKOS). The exact trauma mechanism is still a matter of scientific discussion. The typical femoral and tibial bone bruise patterns may be the result of femoral extension during anteriorly directed acceleration of the tibia (Hashemi 2011), the result of a locked anterior subluxation of the tibia or the following reposition motion in knee flexion. The kinematics associated with ACL related injuries comprise not only the geometry of a motion but also acceleration and velocity. Low knee loading velocity has been shown to be associated with ACL avulsion fractures (Bengston 2011) [102].

## 3 Diagnosis

Paediatric patients with ACL injury typically report an audible snap/pop at the time of injury, followed by rapid onset of hemarthrosis [75]. Consecutive pain and instability typically compromise weight-bearing. However, as children may neglect the injury, prolonged full weight-bearing may be seen [73]. As pain and swelling usually resolve within weeks, acute ACL injuries may be initially overlooked, and chronic ACL injuries first encountered in patients who present with recurrent instability and/or aggravated pain due to secondary meniscal injury. The diagnosis of paediatric ACL injury requires a structured approach due to the presence of open physes and associated injuries [7, 34, 48, 76, 77]. In acute settings, paediatric patients tend to undergo radiographic assessment to visualise bony avulsions which require immediate attention. Clinical evaluation includes inspection, palpation, ROM-assessment and functional tests. The uninjured knee needs to be assessed to define native joint characteristics. Inspection includes assessment of gait-pattern, baseline alignment and leg-length discrepancy, muscle atrophy, kinematics, ROM and contour. Palpation may confirm the presence and degree of effusion as well as reveal relevant musculoskeletal pathology. A positive suprapatellar fluctuation sign may indicate a subtle effusion, previously undetected during inspection. Palpation of joint lines and collateral ligaments may indicate associated meniscus and ligament injury. Functional tests include the Lachman test and pivot-shift test for the assessment of multi-planar stability. Both tests are associated with low reliability in the conscious patient [118]. Standard imaging includes 3 plane radiographs to identify bony avulsions, physeal injuries as well as osteochondral fractures. Baseline leg-length discrepancy and angular deformity may be quantified with standing anteroposterior long-leg radiographs (Shifflett 2016). In addition, the biological age of the patient and geometrical features of the knee are assessed. MRI assessment is used to secure the diagnosis, exclude concomitant meniscal, cartilage and ligamentous injuries and assess maturity and physeal status. Direct signs of ACL injury on MRI include abnormal ligament course, abnormal intensity as well as ligament discontinuity. The most common indirect signs of ACL rupture include typical bone bruise patterns, abnormal PCL angle, anterior tibial displacement, posterior subluxed lateral meniscus as well as lateral femoral notch sign [72]. Additional oblique and 3D imaging typically improve the detection rate of ligament abnormalities. A central aspect in the treatment of paediatric ACL injuries is maturity assessment based on the fact that the risk of growth deformity is inversely proportional to the remaining growth potential. Maturity assessment affects the timing of ACLR and in special cases, non-operative treatment may be indicated until physes have closed. MRI, Tanner staging and non-dominant-hand PA radiographs are currently used to estimate the skeletal age (Zerin 1991; Acheson 1963; Heyworth 2013). Peak growth velocity may be derived from Tanner staging (Granados 2015). MRI assessment may be used for initial assessment of biological age through knee bone age milestones including ossification of the tibial tubercle apophysis [87]. In girls, the tibial tubercle apophysis is typically non-ossified until the age of 10, incompletely ossified displaying a physiological fissure by the age of 11, and completely ossified by the age of 12. In boys, the tubercle apophysis is typically non-ossified until the age of 12, partially ossified displaying a physiological fissure by the age of 13, and completely ossified by the age of 14 (Fig. 1). Postoperative assessment of the patient in order to identify and manage eventual growth disturbance is strongly recommended. Anatomic risk factors associated with ACL injury such as increased anterior pelvic tilt, increased femoral anteversion, intercondylar notch width, femoral condyle ratio as well as increased posterior tibial slope should be assessed [1].

## 4 Management Strategies and Indications

There is currently no consensus on the optimal treatment strategy of paediatric ACL injuries [47, 49, 59, 108, 110]. Even though a growing body of evidence supports early ACLR for patients with recurrent instability as the treatment of choice [41], conservative treatment is regarded as viable treatment option [123]. As a result, the current treatment algorithm is based on individual and thorough patient assessment including knee status and associated intra-articular injuries which require immediate attention, skeletal maturity, patient demands as well as psychological factors [10, 35, 89, 90, 105]. In cases in which surgical treatment is delayed until skeletal maturity, patients and their parents need to be aware of the risk of consecutive meniscal and cartilage injury, especially in the setting of recurrent severe instability [49]. On the other hand, even though paediatric ACLR is associated with satisfactory

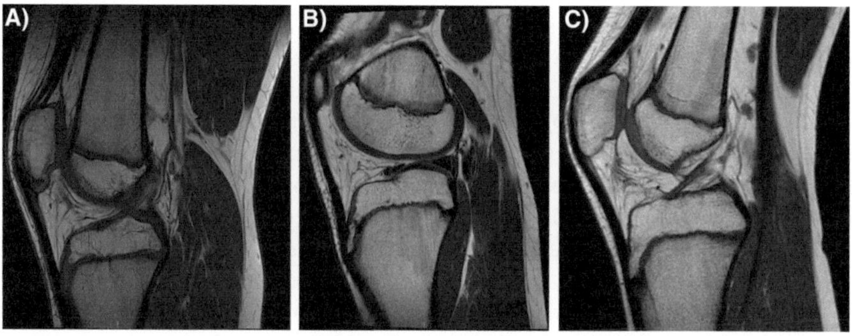


**Fig. 1** MRI based assessment of knee bone age milestones according to Meza et al. [87]. A) Until the age of 10 years for girls and 12 years for boys, the tibial tubercle apophysis is typically non-ossified. B) By the age of 11 years for girls and 13 years for boys, the tibial tubercle apophysis is typically incompletely ossified displaying a physiological fissure. C) By the age of 12 years for girls and 14 years for boys, the tibial tubercle apophysis is completely ossified

results, a significant risk of re-injury and further surgical intervention needs to be considered. In accordance with current paediatric ACL injury treatment algorithms, non-operative treatment is indicated for patients with incomplete ACL tears without significant instability. Non-operative treatment can be summarised by the acronym ABC, **A**ctivity modification, **B**racing and Continuous/**C**ontrolled rehabilitation. Close follow-ups are recommended in order to identify and manage consecutive meniscal and cartilage injury. Bracing without activity restriction has been shown to be associated with increased risk of consecutive meniscal damage and recurrent instability [46]. Non-displaced and minimally displaced tibial eminence fractures may be treated conservatively in an above knee cast in 10–20 degrees of flexion. Aspiration of hemarthrosis has been shown to facilitate reduction of displaced tibial eminence fractures. The current indications for surgery comprise instability impeding sports participation and/or daily living, concomitant injuries which require immediate intervention as well as multi-ligament injury. The timing of ACLR is dependent on several factors including skeletal maturity, the biological/inflammatory status of knee as well as relevant concomitant injury. As distal femoral and proximal tibial physes account for most of the lower-leg-extremity growth, careful consideration of the surgical technique is recommended. Growth under 1 cm in each limb segment can be expected after the age of 13 years in girls, and 14 years in boys (Kelly 2008). Before these ages reconstructive surgery should follow considerations to avoid or minimise physeal damage. The surgical approach to paediatric ACLR can be simplified into physeal sparing, partially transphyseal and transphyseal techniques. The younger the patient, the less physeal-compromising approach must be chosen based on the reciprocal association of remaining growth and potential risk of growth deformity (Seil 2017). In patients younger than 8 years, an intra-articular, extra-physeal approach is a commonly recommended [58, 88]. For the physeal sparing ITB autograft reconstruction an ITB-strip is mobilised while retaining its insertion at Gerdy's tubercle. The graft is brought through the knee, led over-the-top-position and passed anteriorly under the intermeniscal ligament. The graft is then sutured to the periosteum of the femur and tibia. Satisfactory biomechanical and clinical outcomes have been reported in the literature, although the non-anatomic nature of the procedure has been highlighted. In patients of 10 years of age with sufficient epiphyseal maturity to contain sockets, an all-epiphyseal approach may be performed (McCarthy 2012) [4, 40, 71]. A free graft is harvested, in special cases from one of the parents, and sockets are established within the epiphysis. Satisfactory outcomes are typically reported, however, also limb-length and angular deformity requiring surgical correction [57]. In addition, an acute graft angle associated with the procedure may induce increased graft strain and graft failure risk. In patients of 12 years of age, a partially transphyseal approach may be performed ([29]; Lo 1997). While the femoral socket is established within the epiphysis or physis-sparing through the over-the-top position, a vertical and central tibial tunnel is created crossing the physis. Length and angular deformity are typically rare, but re-rupture rates of up to 25% have been reported. In patients of 14 years of age, a transphyseal approach may be performed [25]. Intra-operative imaging is not required. Small diameter tunnels, vertical graft orientation, appropriate graft tension and minimal hardware across the lateral distal femoral physis are among recommended principles. A tripled or quadrupled hamstring tendon with adjustable suspensory fixation on both ends may be used in these cases. BTB grafts must be avoided based on physeal bony ingrowth of the bone plugs and risk of premature physeal arrest [41]. As development of focal physeal disruption following transphyseal ACLR has been shown to occur in 11.6% of the patients without a perceived clinical growth disturbance, transphyseal ACLR should be avoided in patients with substantial remaining growth [124]. There is currently no consensus on rehabilitation following paediatric ACLR. Current rehabilitation protocols are based on adult rehabilitation with specific alterations based on the fact that children display a developing neuromuscular system with unique kinematics, e.g. increased dynamic valgus compared to adults. In addition, while the biological healing response is thought to be improved in children compared to adults, children typically require more time to recover strength and neuromuscular functions (Tang 2023) [13]. Delaying RTS has been shown to reduce re-rupture rates but has also been associated with compromised ROM.

## 5 Growth Plates and Growth Disturbance

Growth abnormalities following ACLR are the result of direct or indirect growth plate tissue influence and can be divided into three categories: Overgrowth, growth arrest and decelerated growth. Overgrowth is caused by local hyper-vascularisation and consecutive stimulation of the physeal growth process, mainly observed in very young children. Growth arrest is typically the result of direct growth plate tissue injury and consecutive formation of a bony bridge. Animal studies suggest that removing more than 4% of the tibial, and more than 7% of the femoral area of the physeal plate is associated with increased risk of growth disturbance (Maekela 1988; Janarv 1998)

[117]. As a rule, removing as little physeal tissue as possible during ACLR is typically recommended, e.g. through small diameter reamers and a vertical tunnel trajectory. However, also physeal sparing techniques have been associated with growth disturbance. Excessive preparation of the over-the-top position for better graft adhesion has been shown to increase the risk of malalignment based on damage of perichondral structures. Decelerated growth is based on the Hueter-Volkmann principle, i.e. growth deceleration based on increased growth plate pressure [44]. As a result, the implantation of a graft per se may induce growth abnormalities through increased tension known as the teno-epiphysiodese effect. In transphyseal approaches, further surgical principles regarding growth plates need to be considered. The risk of a growth deformity is inversely proportional to the remaining growth potential. Excessive graft tension and hardware-physis contact should be avoided. The location of the injury has implications for further deformity. While central growth plate injury leads to symmetric shortening, peripheral growth plate injury leads to axial deformity (Seil SB II). Growth plate injury induced through the femoral tunnel may induce a deformity in valgus and flexion based on the posterolateral location. Growth plate injury induced through the tibial tunnel may lead to genu recurvatum, especially in too anteriorly placed tunnels and tibial tubercle apophyseal arrest (Seil SB I) [41]. As only smaller case series have reported on the incidence of growth disturbance following ACL reconstruction [21], the exact incidence of growth disturbance remains unknown and is thought to be underreported. In a meta-analysis by Wong et al. including 1321 knees, growth disturbance was reported in 58 knees [122].

## 6 Results of Paediatric ACL Reconstruction and Surgical Principles

Several studies have reported results of paediatric ACLR [4, 5, 9, 18, 26, 37, 53, 101, 114] but commonly display various limitations such as retrospective design, small sample size, heterogeneity of the surgical procedure, short-term follow-up, lack of RTS assessment, lack of biological age assessment, lack of information regarding management of the physis as well as unvalidated subjective outcome measures. In addition, changing body geometry associated with the maturity process of children and a variable extend of compliance to rehabilitation protocols and activity restriction contribute to the heterogeneity of a given paediatric study population. As a result, reliable evidence on optimal treatment procedures of ACL deficiency is scarce. Several meta-analyses indicate satisfactory results following early and delayed paediatric ACLR in terms of multi-planar knee stability and subjective outcomes. Delayed ACL reconstruction of more than 12 weeks following ACL injury is commonly associated with increased incidence of irreparable meniscus injury [53]. Complication rate is commonly low, and the incidence of growth disturbance is currently thought to correspond to the incidence of septic arthritis following ACLR. As systematic evaluation of potential growth abnormalities is not performed in all cases, the incidence of growth abnormalities is thought to be underreported [121]. Surgical principles have been derived in order to optimise treatment algorithms. Delaying surgery ensures physical and phycological maturation of the patient. Growth plate injury may be avoided but secondary meniscal and cartilage injury must be considered, especially in the unstable knee. The life-long sequelae of an irreparable lateral meniscus injury with rapid onset of OA have to be weighed against the risk of growth disturbance including limb shortening or angular deformity. No surgical procedure completely eliminates the risk of growth disturbance. Technical considerations for tunnel drilling include vertical tunnel trajectory and slower tunnel drilling to avoid thermal damage. The area of physeal-tissue injury increases non-linearly with increasing reamer diameter. A reamer diameter of 8 mm has been shown to remove 2.5% of the physis tissue, while an 11 mm reamer diameter has been shown to remove 7.8% of the physis tissue in specific scenarios. Bone plugs or interference screws placed across the physis may lead to growth arrest. Development of genu recurvatum based on interference screws crossing the physis even in patients close to skeletal maturity has been reported in the literature [104]. Excessive graft tension should be avoided as compressive forces may lead to growth disturbance [38, 39].

## References


1. Aichroth PM, Patel DV, Zorrilla P. The natural history and treatment of rupture of the anterior cruciate ligament in children and adolescents. A prospective review. J Bone Joint Surg Br. 2002;84(1):38–41.
2. Alentorn-Geli E, Myer GD, Silvers HJ, Samitier G, Romero D, Lazaro-Haro C, Cugat R. Prevention of non-contact anterior cruciate ligament injuries in soccer players. Part 2: a review of prevention programs aimed to modify risk factors and to reduce injury rates. Knee Surg Sports Traumatol Arthrosc. 2009;17(8):859–879. https://doi.org/10.1007/s00167-009-0823-z
3. Anderson M, Green WT, Messner MB. Growth and predictions of growth in the lower extremities. J Bone Joint Surg Am. 1963;45:1–14.
4. Anderson AF, Anderson CN. Correlation of meniscal and articular cartilage injuries in children and adolescents with timing of anterior cruciate ligament reconstruction. Am J Sports Med. 2015 Feb;43(2):275–81. https://doi.org/10.1177/0363546514559912. Epub 2014 Dec 12. PMID: 25497145.
5. Anderson AF. Transepiphyseal replacement of the anterior cruciate ligament using quadruple hamstring grafts in skeletally immature patients. J Bone Joint Surg Am. 2004;86-A Suppl 1.
6. Anderson AF. Transepiphyseal replacement of the anterior cruciate ligament in skeletally immature patients. A preliminary report. J Bone Joint Surg Am. 2003;85-A(7):1255–1263.
7. Arbes S, Resinger C, Vecsei V, Nau T. The functional outcome of total tears of the anterior cruciate ligament (ACL) in the skeletally immature patient. Int Orthop. 2007;31(4):471–5. https://doi.org/10.1007/s00264-006-0225-5.
8. Askenberger M, Ekstrom W, Finnbogason T. Occult intraarticular knee injuries in children with hemarthrosis. Am J Sports Med. 2014;42.
9. Astur DC, Aretti JV, Cavalcante ELB, Goes A, Kaleka CC, Debieux P. Pediatric anterior cruciate ligament reruptures are related to lower functional scores at the time of return to activity: a prospective, midterm follow-up study. Orthopaed J Sports Med. 2019;7.
10. Astur DC, Arliani GC, Debieux P, Kaleka CC, Amaro JT, Cohen M. Intraarticular hamstring graft diameter decreases with continuing knee growth after ACL reconstruction with open physes. Knee Surg Sports Traumat Arthrosc. 2016;24.

11. Barrack RL, Bruckner JD, Kneisl J, et al. The outcome of nonoperatively treated complete tears of the anterior cruciate ligament in active young adults. Clin Orthop Relat Res. 1990;259:192–9.
12. Baxter MP. Assessment of normal pediatric knee ligament laxity using the genucom. J Pediatr Orthop. 1988;8(5):546–50.
13. Beck NA, Lawrence JT, Nordin JD, DeFor TA, Tompkins M. ACL tears in school-aged children and adolescents over 20 years. Pediatrics. 2017;139(3). https://doi.org/10.1542/peds.2016-1877.
14. Beischer S, Hamrin Senorski E, Thome C, Samuelsson K, Thome R. Young athletes return too early to knee-strenuous sport, without acceptable knee function after anterior cruciate ligament reconstruction. Knee Surg Sports Traumatol Arthrosc. 2018;26.
15. Bengtson H, Giangarra C. Osteochondral avulsion fracture of the anterior cruciate ligament femoral origin in a 10-year-old child: a case report. J Athl Train. 2011;46(4):451–5.
16. Boden BP, Dean GS, Feagin JA Jr, Garrett WE Jr. Mechanisms of anterior cruciate ligament injury. Orthopedics. 2000;23(6):573–8.
17. Boden BP, Sheehan FT. Mechanism of non-contact ACL injury: OREF Clinical Research Award 2021. J Orthop Res. 2022;40:531–40. https://doi.org/10.1002/jor.25257
18. Bollen S, Pease F, Ehrenraich A, Church S, Skinner J, Williams A. Changes in the four-strand hamstring graft in anterior cruciate ligament reconstruction in the skeletally-immature knee. J Bone Joint Surg Br. 2008;90(4):455–9. https://doi.org/10.1302/0301-620X.90B4.19416.
19. Bonnard C, Fournier J, Babusiaux D, Planchenault M, Bergerault F, de Courtivron B. Physealsparing reconstruction of anterior cruciate ligament tears in children: results of 57 cases using patellar tendon. J Bone Joint Surg Br. 2011;93(4):542–7. https://doi.org/10.1302/0301-620X.93B4.25801.
20. Bonnard C, Chotel F (2007) Knee ligament and meniscal injury in children and adolescents (Article in French). Rev Chir Orthop Reparatrice Appar Mot. 93(6 Suppl):95–139
21. Buller LT, Best MJ, Baraga MG, Kaplan LD. Trends in anterior cruciate ligament reconstruction in the United States. Orthop J Sports Med. 2014;3(1):2325967114563664.
22. Chotel F, Henry J, Seil R, Chouteau J, Moyen B, Bérard J. Growth disturbances without growth arrest after ACL reconstruction in children. Knee Surg Sports Traumatol Arthrosc. 2010;18:1496–500.
23. Chotel F, Seil R. Growth disturbances after transphyseal ACL reconstruction in skeletally immature patients: who is more at risk? Young child or adolescent? J Pediatr Orthop. 2013;33(5):585–586 14.
24. Chotel F, Bonnard C, Accadbled F, et al. Résultats et facteurs pronostiques de la reconstruction du LCA sur genou en croissance. A propos d'une série multicentrique de 102 cas. Rev Chir Orthop Reparatrice Appar Mot. 2007;93:3S131–3S138.
25. Clanton T, DeLee J, Sanders B, Neidre A. Knee ligament injuries in children. J Bone Jt Surg. 1979;61.
26. Cohen M, Ferretti M, Quarteiro M, Marcondes FB, de Hollanda JP, Amaro JT, Abdalla RJ. Transphyseal anterior cruciate ligament reconstruction in patients with open physes. Arthroscopy. 2009;25(8):831–8. https://doi.org/10.1016/j.arthro.2009.01.01.
27. Courvoisier A, Grimaldi M, Plaweski S. Good surgical outcome of transphyseal ACL reconstruction in skeletally immature patients using four-strand hamstring graft. Knee Surg Sports Traumatol Arthrosc. 2011;19(4):588–91. https://doi.org/10.1007/s00167-010-1282-2.
28. DeLee JC, Curtis R. Anterior cruciate ligament insufficiency in children. Clin Orthopaed Relat Res. 1983;172.
29. Dekker TJ, Godin JA, Dale KM, Garrett WE, Taylor DC, Riboh JC. Return to sport after pediatric anterior cruciate ligament reconstruction and its effect on subsequent anterior cruciate ligament injury. J Bone Joint Surg Am. 2017;99.
30. Demange MK, Camanho GL. Nonanatomic anterior cruciate ligament reconstruction with double-stranded semitendinosus grafts in children with open physes: Minimum 15-year follow-up. American Journal of Sports Medicine 2014;42.

31. Dhillon MS, Rangasamy K, Rajnish RK, Gopinathan NR. Paediatric Anterior Cruciate Ligament (ACL) injuries: current concepts review. Indian J Orthop. 2022;56(6):952–62.
32. Dodwell ER, Lamont LE, Green DW, Pan TJ, Marx RG, Lyman S. 20 years of pediatric anterior cruciate ligament reconstruction in New York State. Am J Sports Med. 2014;42(3):675–80 Epub 2014 Jan 29.
33. Dodwell ER, LaMont LE, Green DW, Pan TJ, Marx RG, Lyman S. 20 Years of pediatric anterior cruciate ligament reconstruction in New York State. Am J Sports Med. 2014;42.
34. Domzalski M, Grzelak P, Gabos P. Risk factors for anterior cruciate ligament injury in skeletally immature patients: analysis of intercondylar notch width using magnetic resonance imaging. Int Orthopaed. 2010;34.
35. Duart J, Rigamonti L, Bigoni M, Kocher MS. Pediatric anterior cruciate ligament tears and associated lesions: epidemiology, diagnostic process, and imaging. J Child Orthop. 2023;17(1):4–11.
36. Dumont GD, Hogue GD, Padalecki JR, Okoro N, Wilson PL. Meniscal and chondral injuries associated with pediatric anterior cruciate ligament tears: relationship of treatment time and patientspecific factors. Am J Sports Med. 2012;40(9):2128–33.
37. Dumont GD, Hogue GD, Padalecki JR. Meniscal and chondral injuries associated with pediatric anterior cruciate ligament tears: relationship of treatment time and patient-specific factors. Am J Sports Med. 2012;40.
38. Edwards PH, Grana WA. Anterior cruciate ligament reconstruction in the immature athlete: longterm results of intra-articular reconstruction. Am J Knee Surg. 2001;14(4):232–7.
39. Edwards TB, Greene CC, Baratta RV, et al. The effect of placing a tensioned graft across open growth plates. A gross and histologic analysis. J Bone Joint Surg Am. 2001;83:725–34.
40. Edwards TB, Greene CC, Baratta RV, Zieske A, Willis RB. The effect of placing a tensioned graft across open growth plates. A gross and histologic analysis. J Bone Joint Surg Am. 2001;83-A(5):725–734
41. Fabricant PD, Jones KJ, Delos D, Cordasco FA, Marx RG, Pearle AD, Warren RF, Green DW. Reconstruction of the anterior cruciate ligament in the skeletally immature athlete: a review of current concepts: AAOS exhibit selection. J Bone Joint Surg Am. 2013;95(5): e28. https://doi.org/10.2106/JBJS.L.0077.
42. Fabricant PD, Kocher MS. Management of ACL injuries in children and adolescents. J Bone Joint Surg Am. 2017;99.
43. Ford LT, Key JA. A study of experimental trauma to the distal femoral epiphysis in rabbits. J Bone Joint Surg Am. 1956;38-A(1):84–92.
44. Frosch KH, Habermann F, Fuchs M, Michel A, Junge R, Schmidtmann U, Stürmer KM. Is prolonged ambulatory physical therapy after anterior cruciate ligament-plasty indicated? Comparison of costs and benefi ts. Unfallchirurg. 2001;104(6):513–8.
45. Frosch KH, Preiss A, Giannakos A. Probleme und Komplikationen nach vorderer. Kreuzbandplastik im Wachstumsalter Arthroskopie. 2012;25:260–5.
46. Gornitzky AL, Lott A, Yellin JL, Fabricant PD, Lawrence JT, Ganley TJ. Sport-Specific Yearly Risk and Incidence of Anterior Cruciate Ligament Tears in High School Athletes: A Systematic Review and Meta-analysis. Am J Sports Med. 2016 Oct;44(10):2716–23. https://doi.org/10.1177/0363546515617742. Epub 2015 Dec 11. PMID: 26657853.
47. Graf BK, Lange RH, Fujisaki CK, Landry GL, Saluja RK. Anterior cruciate ligament tears in skeletally immature patients: meniscal pathology at presentation and after attempted conservative treatment. Arthroscopy. 1992;8(2):229–33.
48. Guzzanti V. The natural history and treatment of rupture of the anterior cruciate ligament in children and adolescents. J Bone Joint Surg Br. 2003;85(4):618–619.
49. Guzzanti V, Falciglia F, Stanitski CL. Preoperative evaluation and anterior cruciate ligament reconstruction technique for skeletally immature patients in Tanner stages 2 and 3. Am J Sports Med. 2003;31(6):941–948.
50. Henry J, Chotel F, Chouteau J, Fessy MH, Bérard J, Moyen B. Rupture of the anterior cruciate ligament in children: early reconstruction with open physes or delayed reconstruction to skeletal maturity? Knee Surg Sports Traumatol Arthrosc. 2009;17(7):748–55.

51. Hewett TE, Myer GD, Ford KR, Paterno MV, Quatman CE. Mechanisms, prediction, and prevention of ACL injuries: Cut risk with three sharpened and validated tools. J Orthop Res. 2016 Nov;34(11):1843–55. https://doi.org/10.1002/jor.23414. Epub 2016 Sep 19. PMID: 27612195; PMCID: PMC5505503.
52. Hinton RY, Rivera VR, Pautz MJ, Sponseller PD. Ligamentous laxity of the knee during childhood and adolescence. J Pediatr Orthop 2008;28(2):184. https://doi.org/10.1097/BPO.0b013e3181652120. Hudgens JL, Dahm DL. Treatment of anterior cruciate ligament injury in skeletally immature patients. Int J Pediatr. 2012;2012:932702
53. Hueter C. Anatomische Studien an den Extremitätengelenken Neugeborener und Erwachsener. Virchow Arch. 1862;25:575–99.
54. James EW, Dawkins BJ, Schachne JM, Ganley TJ, Kocher MS; PLUTO Study Group; Anderson CN, Busch MT, Chambers HG, Christino MA, Cordasco FA, Edmonds EW, Green DW, Heyworth BE, Lawrence JTR, Micheli LJ, Milewski MD, Matava MJ, Nepple JJ, Parikh SN, Pennock AT, Perkins CA, Saluan PM, Shea KG, Wall EJ, Willimon SC, Fabricant PD. Early operative versus delayed operative versus nonoperative treatment of pediatric and adolescent anterior cruciate ligament injuries: a systematic review and meta-analysis. Am J Sports Med. 2021;49(14):4008–4017. https://doi.org/10.1177/0363546521990817. Epub 2021 Mar 15. PMID: 33720764.
55. Kannus P, Jarvinen M. Knee ligament injuries in adolescents. Eight year follow-up of conservative management. J Bone Joint Surg Br. 1988;70:772–6.
56. Kercher J, Xerogeanes J, Tannenbaum A, Al-Hakim R, Black JC, Zhao J. Anterior cruciate ligament reconstruction in the skeletally immature: an anatomical study utilizing 3-dimensional magnetic resonance imaging reconstructions. J Pediatr Orthop. 2009;29(2):124–9. https://doi.org/10.1097/BPO.0b013e3181982228.
57. Kim SJ, Chang JH, Kim TW, Jo SB, Oh KS. Anterior cruciate ligament reconstruction with use of a single or double-bundle technique in patients with generalized ligamentous laxity. J Bone Joint Surg Am. 2009;91:257–62.
58. Koch PP, Fucentese SF, Blatter SC. Complications after epiphyseal reconstruction of the anterior cruciate ligament in prepubescent children. Knee Surg Sports Traumatol Arthrosc. 2016;24(9):2736–40 Epub 2014 Oct 26.
59. Kocher MS, Garg S, Micheli LJ. Physeal sparing reconstruction of the anterior cruciate ligament in skeletally immature prepubescent children and adolescents. J Bone Joint Surg Am. 2005;87(11):2371–9. https://doi.org/10.2106/JBJS.D.02802.
60. Kocher MS, Saxon HS, Hovis WD, Hawkins RJ. Management and complications of anterior cruciate ligament injuries in skeletally immature patients: survey of the Herodicus Society and the ACL Study Group. J Pediatr Orthop. 2002;22(4):452–7.
61. Kocher MS, Smith JT, Zoric BJ, Lee B, Micheli LJ. Transphyseal anterior cruciate ligament reconstruction in skeletally immature pubescent adolescents. J Bone Joint Surg Am. 2007;89(12):2632–9. https://doi.org/10.2106/JBJS.F.01560.
62. Kocher MS, Garg S, Micheli LJ. Physeal sparing reconstruction of the anterior cruciate ligament in skeletally immature prepubescent children and adolescents. Surgical technique. J Bone Joint Surg Am. 2006;88(Suppl 1):283–293
63. Koman JD, Sanders JO. Valgus deformity after reconstruction of the anterior cruciate ligament in a skeletally immature patient. A case report. Bone Joint Surg Am. 1999;81:711–5.
64. Kooy CEVW, Jakobsen RB, Fenstad AM, Persson A, Visnes H, Engebretsen L, Ekås GR. Major Increase in Incidence of Pediatric ACL Reconstructions From 2005 to 2021: A Study From the Norwegian Knee Ligament Register. Am J Sports Med. 2023 Sep;51(11):2891–99. https://doi.org/10.1177/03635465231185742. Epub 2023 Jul 27. PMID: 37497771; PMCID: PMC10478322.
65. Kopf S, Schenkengel JP, Wieners G, Starke C, Becker R. No bone tunnel enlargement in patients with open growth plates after transphyseal ACL reconstruction. Knee Surg Sports Traumatol Arthrosc. 2010;18(11):1445–51. https://doi.org/10.1007/s00167-009-1041-4.
66. Kumar S, Ahearne D, Hunt DM. Transphyseal anterior cruciate ligament reconstruction in the skeletally immature: follow-up to a minimum of sixteen years of age. J Bone Joint Surg Am. 2013;95(1): e1. https://doi.org/10.2106/JBJS.K.01707.

67. Kwon JW, Yoon YC, Kim YN, Ahn JH, Choe BK. Which oblique plane is more helpful in diagnosing an anterior cruciate ligament tear? Clin Radiol. 2009;64(3):291–7. https://doi.org/10.1016/j.crad.2008.10.007.
68. Labella CR, Hennrikus W, Hewett TE. Council on Sports Medicine and Fitness, Section On Orthopaedics Anterior cruciate ligament injuries: diagnosis, treatment, and prevention. Pediatrics 2014;133(5). https://doi.org/10.1542/peds.2014-0623
69. Lawrence JT, Argawal N, Ganley TJ. Degeneration of the knee joint in skeletally immature patients with a diagnosis of an anterior cruciate ligament tear: is there harm in delay of treatment? Am J Sports Med. 2011;39(12):2582–7. https://doi.org/10.1177/0363546511420818.
70. Lawrence JT, Argawal N, Ganley TJ. Degeneration of the knee joint in skeletally immature patients with a diagnosis of an anterior cruciate ligament tear: is there harm in delay of treatment? Am J Sports Med. 2011;39(12):2582–7.
71. Lawrence JT, Bowers AL, Belding J, Cody SR, Ganley TJ. All-epiphyseal anterior cruciate ligament reconstruction in skeletally immature patients. Clin Orthop Relat Res. 2010;468(7):1971–7. https://doi.org/10.1007/s11999-010-1255-2.
72. Lee K, Siegel MJ, Lau DM, Hildebolt CF, Matava MJ. Anterior cruciate ligament tears: MR imagingbased diagnosis in a pediatric population. Radiology. 1999;213(3):697–704. https://doi.org/10.1148/radiology.213.3.r99dc26697.
73. Lohmander LS, Englund PM, Dahl LL, Roos EM. The long-term consequence of anterior cruciate ligament and meniscus injuries: osteoarthritis. Am J Sports Med. 2007;35(10):1756–69. https://doi.org/10.1177/0363546507307396.
74. Makela EA, Vainionpaa S, Vihtonen K, Mero M, Rokkanen P. The effect of trauma to the lower femoral epiphyseal plate. An experimental study in rabbits. J Bone Joint Surg Br. 1988;70(2):187–191
75. Mall NA, Paletta GA. Pediatric ACL injuries: evaluation and management. Curr Rev Musculoskelet Med. 2013 Jun;6(2):132–40. https://doi.org/10.1007/s12178-013-9169-8. PMID: 23575620; PMCID: PMC3702779.
76. Mall NA, Paletta GA. Pediatric ACL injuries: evaluation and management. Curr Rev Musculoskelet Med. 2013;6(2):132
77. Mall NA, Paletta GA. Pediatric ACL injuries: evaluation and management. Current reviews in musculoskeletal medicine. 2013;6.
78. Manner HM, Radler C, Ganger R, Grill F. Dysplasia of the cruciate ligaments: radiographic assessment and classifi cation. J Bone Joint Surg Am. 2006;88(1):130–7. https://doi.org/10.2106/JBJS.E.00146.
79. Matsushita T, Oka S, Nagamune K, Matsumoto T, Nishizawa Y, Hoshino Y, Kubo S, Kurosaka M, Kuroda R. Differences in knee kinematics between wake and anesthetized patients during the Lachman and Pivot-Shift tests for anterior cruciate ligament defi ciency. Orthop J Sports Med. 2013;1(1). https://doi.org/10.1177/2325967113487855
80. Mauro CS, Irrgang JJ, Williams BA, Harner CD. Loss of extension following anterior cruciate ligament reconstruction: analysis of incidence and etiology using IKDC criteria. Arthroscopy. 2008;24(2):146–53. https://doi.org/10.1016/j.arthro.2007.08.026.
81. McCarroll JR, Shelbourne KD, Porter DA, Rettig AC, Murray S. Patellar tendon graft reconstruction for midsubstance anterior cruciate ligament rupture in junior high school athletes. An algorithm for management. Am J Sports Med. 1994;22(4):478–484
82. McCarroll JR, Shelbourne KD, Patel DV. Anterior cruciate ligament injuries in young athletes. Recommendations for treatment and rehabilitation. Sports Med. 1995;20(2):117–127
83. McConkey MO, Bonasia DE, Amendola A. Pediatric anterior cruciate ligament reconstruction. Curr Rev Musculoskelet Med. 2011;4(2):37–44. https://doi.org/10.1007/s12178-011-9076-9.
84. McIntosh AL, Dahm DL, Stuart MJ. Anterior cruciate ligament reconstruction in the skeletally immature patient. Arthroscopy. 2006;22:1325–30.
85. Mccarroll JR, Rettig AC, Shelbourne KD. Anterior cruciate ligament injuries in the young. 1988

86. Meller R, et al. Hindlimb growth after a transphyseal reconstruction of the anterior cruciate ligament: a study in skeletally immature sheep with wide-open physes. Am J Sports Med. 2008;36(12):2437–43.
87. Meza BC, LaValva SM, Aoyama JT, et al. A novel shorthand approach to knee bone age using MRI: a validation and reliability study. Orthopaed J Sports Med. 2021;9(8). https://doi.org/10.1177/23259671211021582
88. Micheli LJ, Rask B, Gerberg L. Anterior cruciate ligament reconstruction in patients who are prepubescent. Clin Orthop Relat Res. 1999;364:40–7.
89. Millett PJ, Willis AA, Warren RF. Associated injuries in pediatric and adolescent anterior cruciate ligament tears: does a delay in treatment increase the risk of meniscal tear? Arthroscopy. 2002;18(9):955–9.
90. Mizuta H, Kubota K, Shiraishi M, et al. The conservative treatment of complete tears of the anterior cruciate ligament in skeletally immature patients. J Bone Joint Surg Br. 1995;77:890–4.
91. Moksnes H, Engebretsen L, Risberg MA. The current evidence for treatment of ACL injuries in children is low: a systematic review. J Bone Joint Surg Am. 2012;94(12):1112–9.
92. Moksnes H, Engebretsen L, Ris berg MA. Performance-based functional outcome for children 12 years or younger following anterior cruciate ligament injury: a two to nine-year follow-up study. Knee Surg Sports Traumatol Arthrosc. 2008;16(3):214–223.
93. Nakhostine M, Bollen SR, Cross MJ. Reconstruction of mid-substance anterior cruciate rupture in adolescents with open physes. J Pediatr Orthop. 1995;15(3):286–7.
94. Newman JT, Carry PM, Terhune EB, Spruiell M, Heare A, Mayo M, Vidal AF. Delay to Reconstruction of the Adolescent Anterior Cruciate Ligament: The Socioeconomic Impact on Treatment. Orthop J Sports Med. 2014 Aug 28;2(8):2325967114548176. https://doi.org/10.1177/2325967114548176. PMID: 26535358; PMCID: PMC4555578.
95. Nordenvall R, Bahmanyar S, Adami J, Stenros C, Wredmark T, Fellander-Tsai L. A populationbased nationwide study of cruciate ligament injury in Sweden, 2001–2009: incidence, treatment, and sex differences. Am J Sports Med. 2012;40(8):1808–13. https://doi.org/10.1177/0363546512449306.
96. Nwachukwu BU, McFeely ED, Nasreddine A, Udall JH, Finlayson C, Shearer DW, Micheli LJ, Kocher M. Arthrofi brosis after anterior cruciate ligament reconstruction in children and adolescents. J Pediatr Orthop. 2011;31(8):811–7.
97. O'Malley MP, Milewski MD, Solomito MJ, Erwteman AS, Nissen CW. The association of tibial slope and anterior cruciate ligament rupture in skeletally immature patients. Arthroscopy. 2015 Jan;31(1):77–82. https://doi.org/10.1016/j.arthro.2014.07.019. Epub 2014 Sep 16. PMID: 25241295.
98. Pascual-Leone N, Gross PW, Meza BC, Fabricant PD. Techniques in pediatric anterior cruciate ligament reconstruction. Arthroscopy. 2022;38(10):2784–6.
99. Patel NM, Bram JT, Talathi NS, DeFrancesco CJ, Lawrence JTR, Ganley TJ. Which children are at risk for contralateral anterior cruciate ligament injury after ipsilateral reconstruction? J Pediatric Orthopedics. 2020;40.
100. Pennock A, Murphy MM, Wu M. Anterior cruciate ligament reconstruction in skeletally immature patients. Curr Rev Musculoskelet Med. 2016 Dec;9(4):445–53. https://doi.org/10.1007/s12178-016-9367-2. PMID: 27586663; PMCID: PMC5127947.
101. Pennock AT, Johnson KP, Turk RD, Bastrom TP, Chambers HG, Boutelle KE, et al. Transphyseal anterior cruciate ligament reconstruction in the skeletally immature: Quadriceps tendon autograft versus hamstring tendon autograft. Orthopaed J Sports Med. 2019;7.
102. Perugia D, Basiglini L, Vadalà A, et al. Clinical and radiological results of arthroscopically treated tibial spine fractures in childhood. Int Orthopaed. 2009;33:243–248. https://doi.org/10.1007/s00264-008-0697-6
103. Petersen W, Bierke S, Stohr A, Stoffels T, Haner M. A systematic review of transphyseal ACL reconstruction in children and adolescents: comparing the transtibial and independent femoral tunnel drilling techniques. J Exp Orthopaed. 2023;10.

104. Peterson DC, Ayeni OR. Pediatric anterior cruciate ligament reconstruction outcomes. Curr Rev Musculoskelet Med. 2016 Dec;9(4):339–47. https://doi.org/10.1007/s12178-016-9358-3. PMID: 27709485; PMCID: PMC5127938.
105. Preiss A, Brodhun T, Stietencron I, Frosch KH. Rupture of the anterior cruciate ligament in growing children: surgical or conservative treatment? A systematic review. Unfallchirurg. 2012;115(9):848–54.
106. Renström PA. Eight clinical conundrums relating to anterior cruciate ligament (ACL) injury in sport: recent evidence and a personal refl ection. Br J Sports Med. 2013;47(6):367–72.
107. Salzmann GM, Spang JT, Imhoff AB. Doublebundle anterior cruciate ligament reconstruction in a skeletally immature adolescent athlete. Arthroscopy. 2009;25(3):321–4. https://doi.org/10.1016/j.arthro.2008.11.008.
108. Seil R, Kohn D. Ruptures of the anterior cruciate ligament (ACL) during growth. Bull Soc Sci Med Grand Duche Luxemb. 2000;1:39–53.
109. Seil R, Pape D, Kohn D. The risk of growth changes during transphyseal drilling in sheep with open physes. Arthroscopy. 2008;24(7):824–33. https://doi.org/10.1016/j.arthro.2008.02.007.
110. Seil R, Robert H. Complete anterior cruciate ligament tears in children. Rev Chir Orthop Reparatrice Appar Mot. 2004;90(8 Suppl):3S11–3S20.
111. Shaw L, Finch CF. Trends in pediatric and adolescent anterior cruciate ligament injuries in Victoria, Australia 2005–2015. Int J Environ Res Public Health. 2017;14(6).
112. Shea KG, Grimm NL, Belzer JS. Volumetric injury of the distal femoral physis during double-bundle ACL reconstruction in children: a threedimensional study with use of magnetic resonance imaging. J Bone Joint Surg Am. 2011;93(11):1033–8. https://doi.org/10.2106/JBJS.J.01047.
113. Shea KG, Pfeiffer R, Wang JH, Curtin M, Apel PJ. Anterior cruciate ligament injury in pediatric and adolescent soccer players: an analysis of insurance data. J Pediat Orthopaed. 2004;24(6):623–628.
114. Shelbourne KD, Gray T, Wiley BV. Results of transphyseal anterior cruciate ligament reconstruction using patellar tendon autograft in tanner stage 3 or 4 adolescents with clearly open growth plates. Am J Sports Med. 2004;32(5):1218–22. https://doi.org/10.1177/0363546503262169.
115. Slough JM, Hennrikus W, Chang Y. The reliability of tanner staging performed by orthopaedic sports medicine surgeons. Med Sci Sports Exerc. 2013;45(7):1229–34.
116. Sobau C, Ellermann A. Anterior cruciate ligament reconstruction with hamstring tendons in the young. Unfallchirurg. 2004;107:676–9.
117. Stadelmaier DM, Arnoczky SP, Dodds J, Ross H. The effect of drilling and soft tissue grafting across open growth plates. A histologic study. Am J Sports Med. 1995;23(4):431–435.
118. Stanitski CL, Harvell JC, Fu F. Observations on acute knee hemarthrosis in children and adolescents. J Pediatr Orthop. 1993;13(4):506–510. Streich NA, Barié A, Gotterbarm T, Keil M, Schmitt H. Transphyseal reconstruction of the anterior cruciate ligament in prepubescent athletes. Knee Surg Sports Traumatol Arthrosc. 2010;18(11):1481–1486.
119. Strobel MW. Vordere Kreuzbandinsuffi zienz. In: Wirth CJ, Zichner L, Kohn D, editors. Orthopädie und orthopädische Chirurgie. Germany: Georg Thieme Verlag, Stuttgart, 2005. p 263–288.
120. Werner BC, Yang S, Looney AM, Gwathmey FW Jr. Trends in pediatric and adolescent anterior cruciate ligament injury and reconstruction. J Pediatr Orthop. 2016;36(5):447–52.
121. Wong SE, Feeley BT, Pandya NK. Complications After Pediatric ACL Reconstruction: A Meta-analysis. Orthop J Sports Med. 2017 Jul 31;5(7 suppl6):2325967117S00434. https://doi.org/10.1177/2325967117S00434. PMCID: PMC5555510.
122. Wong SE, Feeley BT, Pandya NK. Complications After Pediatric ACL Reconstruction: A Meta-analysis. J Pediatr Orthop. 2019 Sep;39(8):e566–71. https://doi.org/10.1097/BPO.0000000000001075. PMID: 31393290.
123. Woods GW, O'connor DP. Delayed anterior cruciate ligament reconstruction in adolescents with open physes. Am J Sports Med. 2004;32:201–10.

124. Yoo WJ, Kocher MS, Micheli LJ. Growth plate disturbance after transphyseal reconstruction of the anterior cruciate ligament in skeletally immature adolescent patients: an MR imaging study. J Pediatr Orthop. 2011;31(6):691–6. https://doi.org/10.1097/BPO.0b013e3182210952.
125. Zacharias AJ, Whitaker JR, Collofello BS, Wilson BR, Unger RZ, Ireland ML, et al. Secondary injuries after pediatric anterior cruciate ligament reconstruction: a systematic review with quantitative analysis. Am J Sports Med. 2020;18.

# ACL Revision

## 1 Introduction

Advances in surgical technique and refined anatomical and biomechanical understanding of the ACL, as well as the implementation of structured rehabilitation following ACLR have led to an overall percentual decrease of ACL revision rates over the past decades [98]. A recent systematic review including 52.878 patients found a revision rate of 3.14% with a mean follow up of 2.3 years [98]. Data from the Norwegian ACL registry including 24.935 patients found an ACL graft re-rupture rate of 4.9% with a mean follow-up of 8.1 years [118]. However, as the incidence of ACL rupture and consecutive reconstruction is steadily increasing, the absolute number of ACL revision procedures is on the rise [87]. ACL revision is indicated if the patient is unsatisfied with the primary ACLR outcome while intending RTS rather than a change in lifestyle and if the cause of failure can be identified and addressed. High sports and daily activity expectations are of greater importance than age for the indication of revision ACLR, especially in the presence of repairable meniscus injury and absence of significant osteoarthritis [27, 85, 134, 161, 207]. Clinical results of ACL revision are typically less predictable and in general, inferior to primary ACLR as reflected by inferior PROM scores, increased risk of postoperative laxity, graft failure as well as meniscal and chondral degeneration [29]. The reason for ACL failure is multifactorial [20, 96, 146, 154, 181, 207] as several factors modulate and determine the susceptibility to ACL graft failure including surgical technique, anatomy, neuromuscular status, concomitant pathology and every factor which increases the risk of trauma exposure such as young patient age, early RTS as well as elite level of sports [150]. ACLR failures can be defined through more or less well-defined endpoints. Objective endpoints of ACLR failure such as pathologic instrumented laxity and radiologically verified ACL graft discontinuity are more likely to result in revision surgery compared to less-well defined endpoints of ACLR failure such as unsatisfactory PROM scores. As a result, ACL failures based on less-well defined endpoints may be underreported. The currently most frequently observed causes for

 
S. Sauer, *ACL Reconstruction: Current Concepts*,
https://doi.org/10.1007/978-3-031-69000-6_6

ACLR failure are thought to be non-anatomic graft orientation, neglected concomitant pathology, traumatic re-rupture, lower extremity malalignment and biological failure [198, 23]. The approach to ACL revision is typically based on individual assessment of the patient including multiple parameters in agreement with patient expectations. Special approaches need to be considered in the setting of residual rotatory laxity, malalignment as well as increased tibial slope. Revision ACL reconstruction is performed as a one-stage or two-stage procedure dependent on several factors including primary ACL tunnel position and status. Autografts are typically preferred over allografts based on lower re-rupture rates. Currently, an increasing role of LEAP in revision ACLR is observed, albeit clear indications and benefits are still controversially discussed [158].

## 2 Definition of ACL Reconstruction Failure

ACLR failure has currently no universal definition but is defined through various more or less well-defined endpoints. Well-defined endpoints include, pathologic antero-posterior instrumented laxity as well as radiologically verified graft discontinuity. Less well-defined endpoints include low PROM scores and compromised knee function which commonly equate to a symptom-complex of one or more subjective and/or objective findings including instability, pain, swelling, stiffness, abnormal gait cycle, loss of motion, extensor mechanism dysfunction as well as OA related symptoms. Four outcome categories of ACL failure are typically distinguished: Adverse events, PROMS, ACL failure or recurrent ligament disruption as well as clinical measures of knee function and structure [168]. As no clear association between these categories has been established, it is recommended to assess all of these categories for the evaluation of ACLR outcomes. ACL failures as defined by objective criteria are more likely to result in revision surgery compared to ACL failures defined by subjective criteria. As a result, revision rates typically underestimate ACL failure rates and underreport failures based on ill-defined endpoints [65]. In general, defining and concretising patient expectations is of paramount importance as a patient related unsatisfactory result of ACLR is invariably defined as an ACLR failure. Conversely, there is no obligatory association between objective and subjective ACLR failure as patients with postoperative increased instrumented residual laxity may perceive a perfectly functioning knee. The most common reasons for ACLR failure and subsequent ACL revision surgery are thought to be graft failure based on new trauma and/or technical surgical error. However, it remains unknown to what extend biological healing and ligamentization disturbance, low virulent infection, graft elongation as well as attritional processes contribute to ACLR failure. A biological failure may become evident through a new trauma based on ACL insufficiency. The majority of ACL failures are identified within the first 2 years after surgery, partly based on increased level of suspicion. While ACL registries gather substantial objective information, subjective patient related information is typically scarce based on low PROM response rates. As the correlation of clinical tests, functional performance and PROMS is thought to be low, the evaluation of ACLR outcomes is increasingly based on all of the aforementioned measures.

## 3 ACL Reconstruction Failure Mechanism

There is currently no consensus in the literature on the single most common cause of ACLR failure. The majority of studies including a prospective longitudinal study by the MARS group identify new trauma as the single most common cause of ACLR failure, followed by technical error and biological failure. Other authors have identified technical error as the single most common cause of ACLR failure [17, 91, 92]. A combination of causes may be present as it remains unclear to what extend biological healing disturbance as well as suboptimal surgical technique modulate the susceptibility to traumatic or attritional graft re-rupture. Clear thresholds for the definition of technical errors are not well-defined. Failure modes and their percentual distribution have been shown to be dependent on primary graft choice with higher rates of biological failure and infection associated with hamstring grafts compared to BPTB grafts. Hamstring grafts show increased risk of healing disturbance at the tendon-bone interface compared to BPTB grafts. Additional factors affecting the susceptibility to graft re-rupture include young patient age, female gender, the geometry of the knee joint, neuromuscular status, concomitant pathology, increased joint laxity (potentially based on connective tissue diseases) [88] and return to pivoting sports on elite level. Factors affecting the susceptibility to biological failure comprise aggressive or neglected rehabilitation, excessive inflammatory response as well as excessive motion at the graft/bone interface (potentially based on technical error). The effect of NSAID on biological healing is not yet fully elucidated. Factors affecting the risk of technical error comprise compromised surgical notch overview, presence of accessory bony ridges mistaken for the resident's ridge, using the lateral meniscus as a reference for tibial tunnel placement in patients with severe static femoro-tibial displacement, small diameter reamer, unusual notch appearance as well as missing remnants.

### *3.1 Technical Error*

Femoral tunnel malpositioning is thought to be the primary cause of ACLR failure based on technical error [150]. Other causes apart from tunnel malpositioning comprise improper graft choice, inadequate graft preparation, fixation and tensioning. Based on the slide-formed anatomy of the posterior aspect of femoral condyle, distal femoral tunnel placement is commonly associated with posterior tunnel placement (down the slide), and proximal tunnel placement is commonly associated with anterior femoral tunnel placement (up the slide). Proximal femoral tunnel placement is associated with grafts tightening in extension, while distal femoral tunnel placement is associated with grafts tightening in flexion. Vertical femoral tunnel placement is associated with increased rotatory laxity. Anterior tunnel placement is associated with increased risk of graft failure [122]. Non-anatomic graft orientation (further influenced by knee position under graft fixation) may induce graft elongation and predispose the graft to mechanical failure. In revision cases of primary transtibial ACLR, a proximal and anterior femoral tunnel is typically encountered which may be associated with residual rotatory laxity. Since the introduction of transportal ACLR, the majority of femoral tunnels are found to be placed too distal and posterior. Decreased direct fiber coverage in femoral tunnels placed too posterior is thought to result in inferior biomechanical stability and increased risk of ACL graft failure [206]. An emerging body of evidence suggests that isometric graft properties may facilitate biological graft related processes, even though the exact mechanism and role of myofibroblasts in controlling graft tension under the process of graft repopulation remains unknown. In regard to tibial tunnel malpositioning, both too anteriorly and posteriorly placed tunnels are thought to be associated with increased risk of graft failure. Too anteriorly placed tibial tunnels may result in roof-notch impingement and consecutive mechanical graft failure. Too posteriorly placed tibial tunnels create a short and vertical graft construct, which typically tightens in extension. In addition, ACL graft impingement against the PCL may cause mechanical graft elongation [198] or mechanical loss of flexion as well as neuromuscular loss of extension based on the proprioceptive ACL reflex. Two-sided mechanical and neuromuscular loss of motion has been associated with the risk of arthrofibrosis development, especially if persisting pain impedes adequate rehabilitation. Medial or lateral malpositioning of the tibial tunnel may result in impingement and iatrogenic chondral and/or meniscal injury [198]. Even after successful integration of a graft following ACLR, the biomechanical graft properties are inferior to the native ACL. The 4-layered anchor architecture of the direct ACL insertion is typically not restored. Altering tibial cartilage slopes shortly after ACL injury alter joint kinematics and enhance strain on the ACL graft and peripheral stabilizing structures. In addition, compromised neuromuscular status increases the risk of re-injury. As a result, re-injury may not be avoidable in all cases. Technical failure comprises improper graft choice, graft diameter, graft preparation, implantation as well as fixation. In terms of graft choice, allografts are associated with significant increased risk of ACL graft failure in the young population compared to autografts. Regarding autografts, it is believed that BPTB grafts are associated with lower failure rates compared to hamstring grafts, albeit several studies have shown similar outcomes. Current data supports the use of the quadriceps tendon for primary and revision ACLR [7, 54, 77]. Graft size has been shown to be influential in terms of ACL failure risk. A diameter of 8 mm is considered the minimal acceptable graft size as thinner grafts have been associated with increased risk of ACLR failure [112, 116]. It has been hypothesised that graft orientation or direct fiber coverage are the underlying cause for these findings as a 6 mm hamstring graft typically exceeds the tensile strength of a 10 mm BPTB graft. In addition, the lower young modulus of HT grafts compared to other grafts is thought to negatively affect the stability of the tendon-bone interface. The optimal graft tension and knee position for tensioning is still a matter of scientific debate. However, over tensioning the graft in non-anatomic positions at the smallest insertional distance does not allow free ROM, elevates joint contact pressure. Under tensioning the graft may result in residual laxity and subjective instability following primary reconstruction. However, the working principle of myofibroblasts in the maintenance or potential increase in tissue tension under graft-repopulation remains unclear. Several other causes are commonly associated with technical error such as hardware malfunction and protrusion, increased interference screw-tunnel divergence angle, inadequate socket length as well as graft source.

## 3.2 *Traumatic Re-rupture*

The risk of traumatic ACL re-rupture is influenced by a variety of factors, primarily those, that increase the risk of trauma exposure and the likelihood of femoro-tibial subluxation through axial forces. Factors increasing trauma exposure include return to high activity level, pivoting sports, elite level of sports, absence of donor site morbidity, early ACLR, young age [6, 35, 197], as well as high psychological readiness to RTS. While high psychological readiness to RTS increases the risk of trauma exposure, low psychological readiness increases the risk of ACL graft re-rupture following RTS [113]. As a result, both high and low psychological readiness are found to be associated with increased risk of ACL graft failure. Factors increasing the likelihood of femoro-tibial subluxation comprise provocative landing positions (hip flexion, slight knee flexion, planted foot), hip-impingement [8, 132] as well as impaired neuromuscular status. In addition, geometrical factors of the knee have been associated with increased risk of recurrent ACL injury including increased posterior tibial bony slope, increased medial-to-lateral condylar size ratio (enhancing the velocity of rotatory kinematics) [70, 190], lateral condylar size ratio, increased posterior cartilage slope, meniscal slope as well as decreased meniscal bone angle and short middle tibial cartilage slope distance [10, 50, 209]. A stenotic notch has been associated with increased risk of ACL failure. Voluminous osteophytes should be resected and a notch-plasty may be necessary, although regrowth of osteophytes is commonly observed [120, 173]. It is conceivable that a properly fixed graft may undergo successful mid-substance repopulation without sufficient maturation of the graft-bone interface. As a result, ACLR failure may be based on attritional changes at some point in the course of rehabilitation. A significant trauma in the following may then represent a causality of insufficiency of the graft construct. Recently, an emerging body of literature indicates an essential role of LEAP´s in primary ACLR for the reduction of ACL failure rates based on temporary biomechanical stabilising effects which are thought to facilitate biological healing processes and reduce femoro-tibial displacement.

## 3.3 Neglected Pathology

An important and avoidable cause of ACL failure is neglected concomitant pathology. ACL injury is commonly associated with concomitant injuries of the menisci and peripheral stabilising structures [3, 14, 15, 101, 159, 162]. The resulting increase in rotatory laxity alters every-day kinematics and may predispose the ACL graft to mechanical failure (Miniami et al. 2018), [212]. As the lateral tibial cartilage slope undergoes morphometrical changes immediately after ACL injury, the integrity and function of anterolateral stabilising structures may become even more significant in controlling rotatory laxity on steeper slopes. Twenty percent of patients undergoing revision ACLR display significant injury of the posterior lateral meniscal root [31]. The integrity of the lateral posterior root is necessary for force transmission and maintenance of physiological femorotibial contact areas. An insufficient posterior lateral meniscal root is associated with increased rotatory laxity and increased risk of ACLR failure. Posterolateral meniscal root repair is typically associated with satisfactory PROMs and healing rates up to 90%. Conversely, lateral joint space narrowing has been associated with these lesions being left untreated [91, 159, 162, 213]. Ramp lesions are thought to be present in up to 15% of patients with ACL injury and have been associated with increased risk of ACLR failure if left untreated [28, 63]. A high-grade Lachman's exam is thought to predict a ramp lesion of the medial meniscus (Familiari et al. 2024). The meniscus ramp-area is defined as the ligamentous connection between the posterior horn of the medial meniscus and the posteromedial tibial head as well as the posteromedial capsule [31]. The role of semimembranosus-traction in the mechanism of ramp lesions is currently elucidated. Meniscal ramp lesions are defined as injury to the peripheral attachment of the posterior horn of the medial meniscus at the meniscocapsular junction or to the meniscotibial attachment. Recently, the anatomy of the medial meniscus has been revisited and revealed that the 2 posterior meniscal attachments merge at a common attachment on the posterior horn of the medial meniscus. The shared attachment-point of the meniscocapsular and meniscotibial attachments has been validated histologically [31]. In several studies, the differentiation between ramp lesions and vertical longitudinal meniscus injuries has been unclear [171]. As a result, a variable incidence of ramp lesions and controversy regarding beneficial effects of repair procedures are found in the literature [121]. The role of the deep MCL has gained attention in controlling rotatory laxity and both anatomic and non-anatomic repair procedures are currently discussed. Overlooked collateral ligament insufficiency may predispose the ACL graft to significantly increased graft strain and risk of mechanical failure.

## 3.4 Biological Failure

The most underreported cause of ACL failure is thought to be biological failure. The currently limited knowledge on ACL graft healing has been derived from MRI studies, animal studies and in vivo biopsy studies. The two most influential processes of graft healing are mid-substance remodelling and graft-bone interface maturation. Through the process of mid-substance remodelling, the graft is repopulated with mesenchymal stem cells after graft necrosis. Myofibroblasts are thought to control in-situ tension of the graft during the process of repopulation. Excessive inflammation and necrosis, poor cell repopulation and proliferation are thought to be associated with increased risk of graft failure. Increased levels of inflammatory mediators including IL-6 and TNF-alpha have been shown to be associated with lower PROM scores. Following mid-substance remodelling, the weak link of the graft is shifted towards the graft/bone interface. The maturation of the fibrovascular interface to a definite anchor architecture is thought to be necessary for graft survival. However, the 4-layered force attuning direct anchor architecture of the native ACL is typically not restored. Instead, a non-uniform indirect anchor architecture through Sharpey fibres is typically observed. The fibrocartilage layers in the native direct insertion contain glycosaminoglycans (GAG) which are thought to provide tissue elasticity and resistance to tensile, shear and compressive forces. Unloading and immobilisation typically induces chondrocyte apoptosis, decreased chondrocyte proliferation and decreased GAG´s in fibrocartilage layers. The tidemark between the mineralised and unmineralised fibrocartilage layer of the direct insertion is of particular interest as it marks a mechanical boundary which is thought to reduce damage to soft tissues during joint movement. In addition, it marks a nutritious barrier. Mechanical stress is thought to be important for the development of fibrocartilage. Increased level of chondrocytes at the tendon-bone interface may be decisive for the formation of fibrocartilage layers. Appropriate mechanical stress of the tendon-bone interface is thought to be important for maturation and eventual completion of the ACL insertion with fibrocartilage and tidemark. Continuous mechanical stress at the bone-graft interface is thought to induce bone tunnel enlargement. The well-described phenomenon does not seem to correlate with functional outcomes but indicates adverse mechanical and/or biological processes [22, 46, 199]. While graft movement within the tunnel (based on graft orientation and young modulus of the graft) [72, 133] is thought to induce mechanical bone tunnel enlargement, implant degradation is thought to induce biological bone tunnel enlargement [46, 119]. In regard to free tendon grafts, complete ossification of the graft inside the tunnel is typically not observed. As a result, biological enhancement has been advocated in order to improve outcomes of ACLR. However, high-quality clinical studies are needed to verify the advantageous impact of biological modulations on ACLR outcomes. The incidence of graft failure in elite athletes is typically concerningly high, even though elite athletes tend to undergo ACLR by experienced surgeons, followed by optimised rehabilitation programs. A better understanding of the biological process of graft healing is thought to eventually reduce graft failure rates in the future. The most common level of single bundle graft rupture is proximal graft rupture. In the early phase, a graft construct is exposed to forces and torques induced by everyday kinematics. A sufficiently sized, anatomically placed and properly secured graft is fundamental for successful ACLR.

## 4 Clinical Presentation of ACL Reconstruction Failure

Any persistent abnormal knee function following primary ACLR which concerns the patient may be defined as ACLR failure. There is no necessary association between objective and subjective failure. In most cases, ACL failure is based on instability, compromised range of motion and/or persistent pain.

### *4.1 Failure Associated with Instability*

ACL failure associated with instability may comprise residual as well as early or late emerging instability which may be persistent or limited to specific motion patterns. The main reason for early emerging instability is hardware malfunction, insufficient graft fixation, graft pull-out, graft damage, biological graft failure as well as graft elongation. The main reason for late emerging instability is traumatic re-rupture, attritional graft damage, graft elongation once ROM is restored in the course of rehabilitation, insufficient healing of the bone-graft interface and may be facilitated based on underlying mechanisms such as neuromuscular imbalance, increased rotatory laxity, insufficient graft diameter or non-anatomic graft orientation. The main reason for residual rotatory instability is typically based on non-anatomical graft positioning (e.g. vertical grafts) [93], neglected concomitant injury of the anterolateral complex and meniscal root injury. In special cases, secondary addition of a LEAP can be considered. Traumatic re-rupture after the patient has fully recovered may in some cases be regarded as ACL re-injury rather than ACL failure. However, graft re-rupture may be based on several modifiable underlying factors. It is therefore important to rigorously address all possible causes of ACLR failure in order to ensure graft longevity following ACL revision.

### *4.2 Failure Associated with Compromised Range of Motion (ROM)*

Failure due to compromised ROM may comprise a one-sided or a two-sided deficit. A one-sided deficit may be based on non-anatomic graft orientation, arthrogenic muscle inhibition, lack of neuromuscular control as well as concomitant injuries. Two-sided deficits are typically based on excessive inflammatory responses associated with effusion, persistent pain, insufficient remobilisation, CRPS as well as arthrofibrosis. In regard to graft orientation based on tibial tunnel placement, too anteriorly oriented grafts are at risk of roof-notch impingement with consecutive loss of extension or mechanical graft failure. Anteriorly oriented grafts tighten in flexion, while posteriorly oriented grafts tighten in extension [45]. Too posteriorly oriented grafts are at risk of impingement against the PCL with loss of flexion and, based on the activated reflex arc of the PCL, also neuromuscular related loss of extension. In regard to graft orientation based on femoral tunnel placement, too anteriorly oriented grafts may restrict flexion while too posteriorly oriented grafts may restrict extension. The differentiation between mechanical or neuromuscular causes of loss of motion represents a diagnostic challenge. In some cases, graft elongation with restoration of ROM is observed. In other cases, especially in the presence of persistent pain, ROM may remain chronically compromised.

## *4.3 Failure Associated with Pain*

Persisting pain following ACLR is a well-known multifactorial condition. Pain as the primary symptom rarely results in ACL revision surgery. However, re-intervention and even resection of the ACL graft may be necessary in specific scenarios. The cause of significant pain may represent a diagnostic challenge and typically originates from exacerbation of existing pathology including OA, anterior knee pain, musculoskeletal disorders, immunologic diseases, irreparable, conservatively treated or neglected pathology including meniscal and chondral injury, collateral ligament injury and malalignment, pathology directly associated with the surgical intervention including technical error, hardware related problems, meniscectomy, donor site morbidity, patella fracture, quadriceps tendon rupture, nerve injury, CRPS, excessive synovitis as well as low-virulent infection. Even though high level evidence is lacking, a few surgical principles are believed to reduce the risk of ACL failure based on persistent pain. Anterior knee pain is thought to be present in up to 47% of patients following ACLR. Any patellofemoral pathology including osteochondral lesions, patellar instability, trochlea dysplasia, patella alta as well as quadriceps weakness may exacerbate anterior knee pain to a level of subjective failure. In cases of infrapatellar contracture syndrome, a patella baja can be observed and increased contact forces may aggravate anterior knee pain. As BPTB grafts are associated with increased risk of patellofemoral OA, BPTB grafts should be avoided in patients with relevant patellofemoral disorders. In addition, complete closure of the ITB following LEAP should be avoided in patients with patellofemoral disorders. Autografts with patellar bone-plugs should be avoided in patients with hypo-plastic patellae, high BMI, advanced age, diabetes mellitus, osteoporosis and any other factor that may increase the risk of patella fracture peri-operatively or in the course of rehabilitation. Preoperatively compromised ROM is typically associated with loss of motion following ACLR. In these patients, adequately sized grafts in anatomic position without causing impingement is of paramount importance. Too posteriorly placed tibial tunnels create a short vertical graft construct which tightens in extension but impinges against to PCL in flexion. Activation of the neuromuscular reflex arc may further aggravate two-sided loss of motion with impact on the gait cycle and resulting pain. It is important to identify any potential injury or pathologic condition that may induce persistent pain. The treatment strategy is depended on the underlying cause of pain and in many cases, a multidisciplinary approach is recommended.

## 5 Management of ACL Reconstruction Failure

There is currently no comprehensive, all-encompassing algorithm for ACL revision surgery. However, consensus agreements emphasise organised approaches and meticulous planning of ACLR revision surgery with individualised strategies to address the unique complexity of a given case [36, 43, 51, 57, 79, 82, 136].

### *5.1 Surgical Planning*

The planning of ACL revision surgery includes consideration of previous information, present characteristics as well as resulting implications for the future. All relevant information regarding the previous course of treatment is typically reviewed, including information on ACL injury mechanism, pre-injury sporting activities and level of activity, rehabilitation and prevention measures, RTS-timepoint, primary surgery details (including graft choice and dimension, drilling technique, fixation methods and implants), previously treated and neglected concomitant injuries, surgical complications as well as conditions affecting the biomechanics of the affected limb including hip impingement, history of septic arthritis, chronic disorders such as inflammatory related diseases and connective tissue diseases such as Marfan syndrome [167, 186]. Present patient characteristics including age, gender, BMI, smoking [85], current level of activity, current activities of daily living, current symptoms (including pain, swelling, instability, clicking, locking, stiffness, muscle fatigue) and symptom duration as well as current knee and contralateral status are identified. Clinically, several factors need to be assessed including anterior–posterior laxity, rotatory laxity, integrity of the anterolateral and anteromedial complex, medial collateral ligament, lateral collateral ligament, PCL and posterolateral corner, range of motion, alignment, gait cycle, signs of meniscus and cartilage injury, donor site morbidity, biological condition of the knee, hyper-laxity, muscle atrophy, neurovascular status, soft tissue status of the lower limb as well as muscle excursion and strength. Anteroposterior laxity is typically assessed by the Lachman test in 20–30 degrees of knee flexion, either manually or instrumented by means of a rolimeter or KT-1000/2000. Rotatory laxity is typically assessed through the pivot-shift test and the severity of an abrupt shift graded from 0, i.e. absent to 4, i.e. gross. The reliability of the pivot-shift test is controversially discussed and attempts of standardisation have been undertaken in order to improve the reliability of the pivot-shift test [75, 100, 130]. Newer technologies have shown promising results for the quantification of the pivot-shift test but do not yet seem completely feasible in the clinical setting. Lab tests (CRP, ESR, FBC) are recommended. Low-virulent infection and any significant comorbidity need to be ruled out. Radiographs and CT are typically used to assess tunnel position, tunnel-aperture dimension, osteolysis and tunnel widening. Full-length radiographs of the lower limb for assessment of coronal and sagittal plane malalignment are recommended. In addition, lateral, flexion weight-bearing antero-posterior as well as patellofemoral radiographs are recommended for the assessment of OA [16]. TELOS radiography is recommended in the setting of collateral ligament insufficiency for the quantification of potential side-to-side differences [13]. CT 3D reconstruction has been shown to facilitate the assessment of tunnel location, status and dimension [89, 115] (Fig. 1). MRI assessment typically includes evaluation of concomitant structural injury, hardware position, tunnel characteristics, tibial cartilage slopes and geometrical factors affecting the outcome of ACL revision (Fig. 2).

Specific MRI-sequences are useful for the assessment of altered rotational femoro-tibial position and frequently overlooked concomitant injuries including meniscal root injuries. 3D MRI is recommended for assessment of ALC integrity. In terms of implications for the future, the patient should be counselled on indications, advantages and disadvantages of staged revision, additional extra-articular stabilisation, slope correcting osteotomies and expected outcome based on gathered information and present evaluation. The surgical approach including graft choice, bone grafting, LEAP as well as rehabilitation protocols need to be adapted accordingly. Furthermore, patient expectations need to be discussed and realistically attuned. Prior to ACL revision, free range of motion should be established. Arthrofibrosis and infrapatellar contracture syndrome should undergo release procedures and intensive rehabilitation prior to revision procedures. Autografts are typically preferred over allografts based on lower risk of re-rupture and better PROMS, higher RTS rates as well as less instrumented laxity [9].

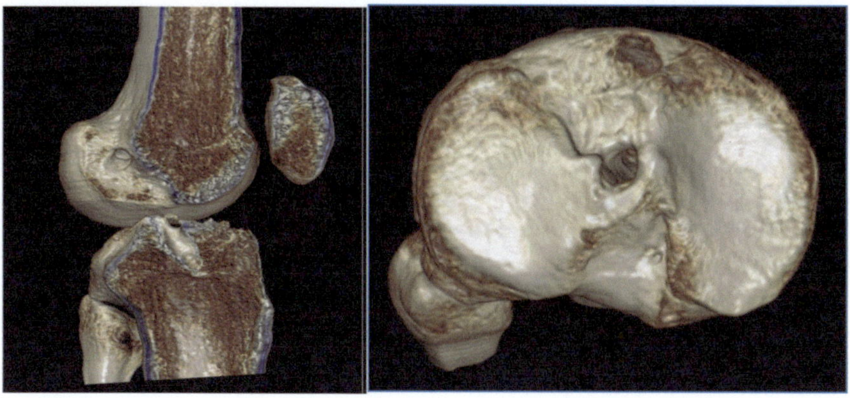

**Fig. 1** 3D CT reconstruction for the assessment of femoral and tibial tunnel position

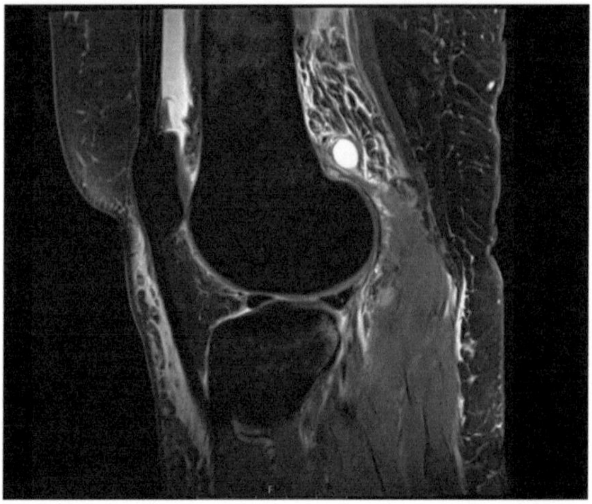

**Fig. 2** MRI assessment of cartilage and meniscal geometry, concomitant pathology and femoro-tibial displacement. The combination of steep lateral posterior tibial cartilage slope, reduced MBA, static femoro-tibial displacement and meniscus injury may be associated with increased dynamic rotatory laxity. Altered rotational femoro-tibial position on MRI has been found to be associated with concomitant MRI determined anterolateral complex (ALC) injury [210]

# 6 Surgical Approach

## *6.1 One Stage Revision*

Global ligamentous integrity and range of motion of the knee should be re-assessed under anaesthesia. If a previously undetected high-grade pivot-shift test is present under anaesthesia, LEAP may be re-considered as a high-grade pivot-shift test represents a risk factor for ACLR failure [3]. The knee is assessed arthroscopically focusing on concomitant injuries and pathology, tunnel position, tunnel dimension and aperture appearance, hardware position and tunnel back-wall integrity. A thorough debridement is recommended in order to clearly visualise graft insertion areas and hardware. A cyclops formation, a hypertrophic scar in the notch and residual graft material is resected. Hardware is removed if impeding the planned procedure or potentially influencing biological healing processes. Unnecessary hardware removal should be avoided to secure biomechanical pull-out strength of the construct. A notchplasty is recommended in cases of a narrow notch compromising visual overview. Following initial inspection and preparation, reassessment of the planned procedure is recommended, and adjustments are performed accordingly. Any concern regarding the practicability of single stage revision should lead to conversion to two-staged revision. Even though a clear cut-off value for two stage revision depended on tunnel dimension has not been agreed upon in the literature, tunnels of 16 mm diameter and beyond rarely undergo single stage revision [148]. However, allograft bone cylinders used to compensate bone loss and secure sufficient graft fixation have shown promising results even in severe tunnel widening. Aperture tunnel dimension exceeds tunnel dimension based on the oblique surface contact of the reamer. The femoral tunnel is inspected, and the intended revision-tunnel position is defined in accordance with the intended graft fixation method. Grafts which are fixed with suspensory fixation have full circumferential tunnel contact while graft fixed with interference screws are pressed eccentrically against the tunnel wall. In cortical suspension fixation, smaller screws can be used to position the graft within the tunnel. Even though there is conflicting evidence regarding the overall most favourable femoral tunnel position, the currently most advisable positions are the centre of the ACL insertion area and the direct insertion area of the AM bundle. Newer research emphasises the biomechanical advantage of direct fibre coverage, located adjacent to the resident's ridge, extending approximately 5 mm posteriorly. In some cases, the centre of the ACL insertion area does not lie within the direct insertion area. In the distal–proximal dimension, the AM bundle position is thought to be associated with minimal length changes of the graft during range of motion which is thought to facilitate biological healing processes including myofibroblast based in-situ tension maintenance of the graft during repopulation. It has been hypothesised that LEAP may dynamically support the graft towards extension. A tunnel located on the direct insertion of the AM bundle is typically intersected by a tangent from the posterior cartilage/bone junction in line with the Blumensaat's line, while being located as proximal as possible on the medial wall of the femoral condyle. Fluoroscopy represents a reliable method for consistent tunnel placement. Once the new tunnel position is defined, one of four scenarios based on the overlapping area with the preexisting tunnel is typically present: a) total or near-total overlapping, i.e. completely correct, b) over 50% of overlapping area, i.e. incompletely correct c) under 50% of overlapping area, i.e. incompletely incorrect, d) no overlapping, i.e. completely incorrect. Total or near-total overlapping tunnels are typically re-used if suitable for graft fixation. If any concern arises with bone tunnel wall integrity, cortical fixation methods are advisable. Hardware is removed and tunnels are debrided by consecutive drilling until fresh cancellous bone is visible. Bone Tunnels exceeding 16 mm diameter tend to undergo staged revision. Similarly, in cases in which low-virulent infection is assumed, all hardware should be removed and conversion to two-stage revision is typically recommended. In tunnels with over 50% of overlapping area (b, a decision must be made whether the tunnel should be drilled parallel to the preexisting tunnel, creating an oval but parallel formation or whether the new tunnel should be drilled non-parallel, creating tunnel overlap at the aperture. In parallel tunnels and ovoid aperture formations, a BTB-graft with a bone plug fixed with an oversized screw is recommended. If any concern with the integrity of the posterior bone wall is assumed, non-parallel tunnels can be established, and cortical suspension devices can be used. In tunnels with under 50% of overlapping area (c, it is advisable to remove absorbable implants to avoid chronic inflammatory tunnel reactions. The preexisting tunnel is then filled with bone plugs, allograft bone dowels) [44], bone screws, PEEK-screws or other suitable material such as fast setting bone substitutes or through impaction of bone [142, 157]. The new tunnel can then then be drilled with minor elimination of tunnel substitutes [41]. In tunnels with no coverage (d), hardware is usually left in situ if non-absorbable. It must be ensured that new tunnels are debrided and suitable for sufficient new graft fixation and for formation and maturation of a reliable bone-graft interface. In cases of severe tunnel widening, a two-stage procedure is commonly recommended. However, auto and allograft bone cylinders or stacked screws [135, 136] in combination with grafts with bone blocks and oversized screws have shown promising results even in cases with severe tunnel widening [38]. Recently, a trend towards LEAP in all revision cases has been observed. The ITB graft is typically attached to the femur in a separate tunnel, inserted into an outside-in ACL tunnel in conjunction with the ACL graft, fixed with suture anchors or looped around the LCL and sutured back to itself, e.g. Cocker-Arnold procedure. The over-the-top procedure should be considered in special cases and is commonly associated with satisfactory functional outcomes. A small opening is hereby created in the intermuscular septum. A tract is created through blunt dissection at the posterolateral aspect of the intercondylar notch [198]. The area is decorticated, creating a bleeding cancellous channel. The graft is led into the groove through the septal hiatus and secured with a staple. A versatile option for reaming the femoral tunnel is through the outside-in technique. The technique requires an accessory lateral incision but enables free tunnel orientation towards the intended aperture location. In addition, the risk of tunnel convergence with LEAP can be minimised. In regard to tunnel position, the fixation method must be considered. Decisive for the biomechanical properties of the graft is not tunnel position but location of the graft within the tunnel after fixation. As interference screws eccentrically compress the graft to the tunnel wall, the centre of the tunnel must be created accordingly. If a BTB graft is used and the bone-plug is planned to cover the direct ACL insertion (with a screw "above" the graft), the centre of the tunnel must be located "above" the lateral intercondylar ridge and outside the anatomical ACL insertion area. Regarding tibial tunnel assessment, complete incorrect tunnel location is seldom. Most tunnels are placed too posteriorly, associated with a short graft construct tightening in extension, eventually inducing graft elongation or mechanical failure. Impingement against the PCL may lead to loss of flexion and further aggravate loss of extension through a neuromuscular reflex arc. Anterior graft orientation based on too anteriorly placed tibial tunnels is associated with roof notch impingement and loss of extension. As the graft construct may tighten in flexion, also loss of flexion may be present. The lateral meniscus is not a reliable landmark for tibial tunnel placement, especially in cases with significant static femoro-tibial displacement. Other landmarks may be identified including the Parson's knob in order to ensure correct tibial tunnel placement. The anterior and posterior roots of the lateral meniscus are at danger of iatrogenic injury under the process of reaming. Cases in which the posterior meniscal root has been accidentally eliminated by reaming have been described in the literature and are probably underreported. However, a complete-incorrect tibial tunnel position is rare. One of the main challenges in regard to tibial tunnels represent substantial tunnel enlargement with posterior and lateral located tibial tunnels. In these cases, a new tunnel with anatomic tunnel aperture location is created, followed by insertion of an interference screw to keep the graft in an anatomic position. Care must be taken not to undermine the tibial plateau or to increase the risk of anterior tibial fracture. Significant bone tunnel enlargement should lead to conversion to two-stage revision. Tibial tunnels with anatomical aperture can be re-used or a different tunnel direction with the same aperture can be created [56]. The new tunnel aperture can be positioned more anteriorly or posteriorly by eccentric reaming. An interference screw is then placed diametral to the reamed aperture expansion for anatomic graft position within the tunnel. It is advisable to remove absorbable screws in order to avoid biological processes which may aggravate bone resorption. Back-up fixation is recommended in the presence of compromised bone quality. The use of straight reamers is recommended to minimise drill drifting commonly associated with acorn type reamers. The bone walls are refreshed and sclerotic bone and eventual cicatricial tissue from the bone-graft interface is removed. Bone tunnels from previous procedures including transtibial pull-out root repairs must be considered, especially if malpositioned. It is advisable to manage and complete all necessary procedures before graft harvest as complications which require conversion to two-stage revision cannot always be foreseen. A possible algorithm for ACL revision. One possible algorithm for revision ACL reconstruction based on primary tunnel location and status is shown in Fig. 3.

## *6.2 Graft Choice*

To date, there is no consensus on optimal graft choice in revision ACLR, partially based on individual graft availability dependent on the primary procedure and special circumstances of a given case. Most commonly used autografts include ipsilateral or contralateral [47, 95, 160] gracilis/semitendinosus, quadriceps tendon and BPTB grafts. Allografts with oversized bone blocks (e.g. BPTB, achilles tendon, quadriceps tendon) are of interest in large diameter tunnels and bone loss. Autografts are typically preferred over allografts as autografts have been shown to be associated with improved activity function [84] and PROMs as well as decreases risk of graft re-rupture when compared to allografts [9, 90]. Equivalent failure rates of allografts compared to autografts have been reported for non-irradiated allografts [25]. BPTB-grafts are of interest for compensation of large bony defects [52, 172, 144] and oversized tibial bone blocks are a viable grafts option but are associated with increased risk of proximal tibial fracture. Synthetic grafts are typically avoided based on unsatisfactory results and excessive synovitis [39, 57]. BPTB grafts are typically associated with lower risk of graft failure and better instrumented laxity compared to hamstring autografts but are associated with increased risk of anterior knee pain [110, 211]. However, in terms of graft failure, several studies indicate similar outcomes when comparing BPTB-grafts and hamstring grafts [140]. Quadriceps autograft is thought to represent a viable graft option for primary and revision ACLR based on similar graft re-rupture rates, functional outcomes and donor site morbidity when compared to hamstring grafts, and significantly less donor site morbidity when compared to

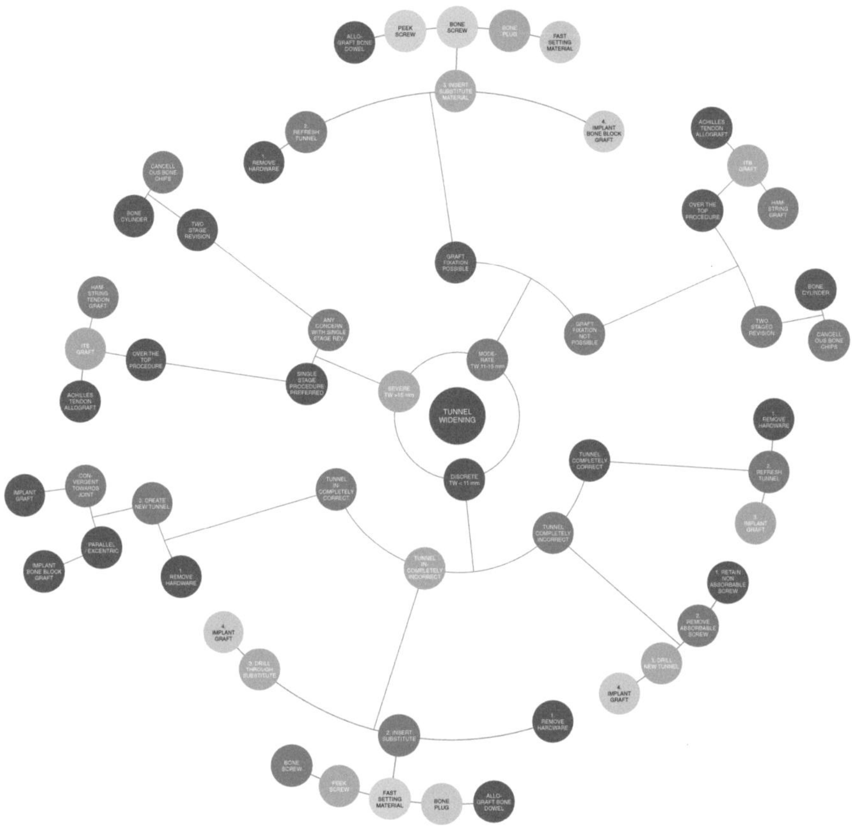


**Fig. 3** Algorithm for revision ACL reconstruction based on primary tunnel location and status

BPTB grafts [7, 9]. Fresh frozen allografts are preferred over irradiated allografts based on lower risk of failure and adverse immunologic response (Toyama et al. 1996) [143, 156]. However, the concern of potential viral and bacterial contamination remains [117]. In double bundle revision, AM tunnels are typically revised while PL tunnels are filled with substituted material. When harvesting contralateral grafts, unless two-sided bone-blocks are needed, it is recommended to harvest HT grafts associated with lower donor site morbidity compared to BPTB [83].

## 6.3 *Two Stage Revision*

Two stage revision is associated with lower re-revision rates and risk of clinical failure compared to single stage revision [30]. However, the risk of chondral and meniscal degeneration as well as early structural changes of cartilage slopes associated with

ACL insufficiency must be considered [37, 136]. Two stage revision may represent a planned procedure or the result of intra-operative conversion from single-stage to two-stage revision based on several factors including primary tunnel status and location, compromised ROM, potential low-virulent infection, concomitant pathology, malalignment, meniscal and/or ligamentous insufficiency [24, 42, 126]. A thorough clinical exam under anaesthesia is recommended [87]. Under primary arthroscopic examination, infection needs to be ruled out. Assessment and treatment of concomitant injuries that require intervention are typically performed. Chondral and meniscal pathology may be more complex as suggested on MRI. Graft remnants are removed in order to adequately inspect preexisting tunnels and hardware is removed. Tunnels are refreshed through consecutive reaming and/or a fine drill. Curettage and other suitable instruments are used to debride the tunnel completely from remnants of the bone-graft interface until fresh cancellous bone is visible. Cylindrical bone autografts from the tibia or iliac crest are typically preferred over allograft cancellous chips based on superior biological response. Both the insertion of cancellous chips and bone dowels are carefully impacted under direct visualisation. Bone dowels should exceed the tunnel diameter by 1 mm for press-fit fixation and are typically transferred by the tube system used for harvesting or may be guided over a guide wire in special cases. Previous concerns with stability of bone graft materials have been resolved based on evidence of early neovascularization of the bone graft and consecutive sufficient stability through strong biologic activity. CT based assessment of bone integration 3 months following bone grafting is recommended. Approximately 6 months after the first stage, and following bony integration, the second stage is performed in analogy to primary ACLR. Fluoroscopy for optimal tunnel placement of ACLR and concomitant procedures is recommended. The main advantage of two-staged revision is the straightforwardness of the second stage [52]. However, the second stage should not be delayed more than 6 months in order to minimise the risk of meniscal and cartilage degeneration [45]. Complications of two stage revision are probably underreported and comprise donor-site morbidity from bone harvest locations, nerve injury as well as blow out. Under bone grafting with cancellous allograft chips in the femoral tunnel, gravity and fluid flow may lead to back-fall of the bone chips into the joint. Careful impaction with a tube system is recommended. When grafting with autograft or allograft bone plugs, direct visualisation of the impaction is recommended, in order to ensure that the graft advances and ends flush with the socket aperture without tunnel blow out.

## 7 Postoperative Rehabilitation

Rehabilitation after revision ACLR typically follows a similar protocol to primary ACLR, albeit several factors may require adjustments of the rehabilitation sequence including bone quality and fixation strength, tendency to excessive inflammatory response, concurrent procedures, concomitant pathology and chronic diseases, psychological status as well as muscle status. In general, a slower progression towards

RTS and high load muscular strength training, especially after 2 two-stage revision is recommended. Full compliance to rehabilitation programs is associated with higher rates of RTS. Systematic assessment of potential psychological distress, fear avoidance behaviour as well as low perceived self-efficacy has been shown to be a significant aspect of rehabilitation [115, 116]. Bracing is typically avoided as no clear beneficial effect are observed [11, 204], unless needed after concurrent procedures that require ROM restriction, e.g. meniscal root repair and collateral ligament reconstruction [11]. The effects of dynamic bracing on ACL graft healing and ALC integrity are currently elucidated. In general, rehabilitation following revision ACLR is typically more restrictive compared to primary ACLR based on increased prevalence of concomitant procedures, compromised bone quality and fixation stability.

## 8 Concurrent Procedures

Most commonly performed concurrent procedures in the setting of revision ACLR comprise osteotomies, meniscal and cartilage surgery as well as LEAP. Varus/valgus malalignment of the lower limb has been found to be associated with increased risk of ACL graft failure based on increased graft strain [123, 174]. Osteotomies to correct coronal malalignment are typically recommended in patients with varus or valgus deviation exceeding 5° accompanied by early OA as well as significant cartilage injury and/or symptomatic meniscal defects in patients with varus or valgus deviation associated with ligamentous insufficiency [14, 69]. Coronal plane malalignment is typically corrected through HTO´s where the mechanical axis is restored through the apex of the lateral tibial eminence (Pache) [151]. The systematic assessment of posterior tibial slope in all revision cases is currently recommended [10, 50] as posterior tibial slope has been shown to be associated with increased risk of AP laxity and ACL failure [149, 209]. Even though no clear cut-off value for the indication of slope correcting osteotomies has been established, most authors consider a slope correcting osteotomy in cases of posterior tibial slope exceeding values of 12 degrees on lateral radiographs [33]. Slope correcting osteotomies aim to correct bony slope to values of 6 degrees, hereby decreasing unphysiological ACL graft forces [78] and rotatory velocity. Hyperextension and PCL graft strain are typically enhanced by slope correcting osteotomies, wherefore PCL insufficiency and hyperextension exceeding 5 degrees are thought to represent relative contra-indications for slope correcting osteotomies. Recently, the assessment of cartilage slopes has gain scientific attention as cartilage slopes are biomechanically decisive. As cartilage slopes increase significantly short after ACL injury, the assessment of cartilage slopes may indicate the necessity of minimising internal tibial rotation through LEAP. As both tibial translation and internal tibial rotation shift the lateral femoro-tibial contact area from the middle cartilage slope towards the steeper posterior cartilage slope of the lateral tibial plateau, lateral meniscal root injuries (increased rotation) and medial meniscal root injuries (increased translation) [101] potentiate the impact of tibial slope on graft strain and the risk of femoro-tibial subluxation (Dejour et al. 2018).

Meniscal insufficiency has been found to significantly increase the risk ACL failure [138]. As a result, rigorous assessment and repair of meniscal injuries is recommended. While the necessity and beneficial effect of posterior meniscal tissue and root repair has been widely agreed upon in the literature, the necessity and beneficial effects of *true* ramp-area-disruption repair (repair of connective tissue) is still controversially discussed. The prevalence of ramp lesions is thought to be high [28]. In the setting of substantial meniscal loss, meniscal transplantation should be considered. Recently, the role of LEAP in revision ACLR has gained significant attention. Several studies have shown a decrease in failure rates following combined ACLR + LEAP compared to isolated ACLR. The combination of ACLR + LEAP should be considered in young active athletes involved in pivoting sports with increased joint laxity (e.g. high-grade pivot-shift, grad II-III anteroposterior instability and/or hyperlaxity) [58, 66].

## 9 Results and Complications Following Revision ACL Reconstruction

While objective outcomes following revision ACLR have been shown to comparable to primary ACLR in most cases, subjective outcomes tend to be inferior when compared to primary ACLR [36]. One reason for this finding is thought to be based on accumulated concomitant pathology. The majority of comparative studies indicate increased prevalence and severity of chondral and meniscal pathology with implications for overall knee function in patients undergoing revision ACLR compared to patients undergoing primary ACLR [203]. As patients with significant cartilage pathology and resulting pain are less likely to undergo revision ACLR, the incidence and severity of concomitant cartilage pathology in patients undergoing revision ACLR is probably underreported. The discrepancy between objective and subjective postoperative outcome is thought to be more distinct in patients undergoing revision ACLR compared to primary ACLR. While objective findings are comparable between primary and revision ACLR including instrumented laxity and results of the pivot-shift test, PROM scores are typically lower in patients undergoing ACLR revision compared to patients undergoing primary ACLR. A multi-centre study by the MOON group revealed lower IKDC scores as well as lower KOOS pain, sports/recreation and QOL sub-scales of patients undergoing revision ACLR compared to patients undergoing primary ACLR. Accordingly, registries reveal overall inferior PROMS of patients undergoing revision ACLR compared to patients undergoing primary ACLR at 1 year follow up. Even though patients undergoing revision ACLR show improved Lysholm score and Tegner-activity-level postoperatively, approximately one-third of the patients consider their knee abnormal or severely abnormal in terms of IKDC. Nevertheless, patients undergoing ACL revision have similar RTS rates compared to patients undergoing primary ACLR, albeit chances of returning to the same level of sport are typically lower in patients undergoing revision ACLR when compared to patients undergoing primary ACLR. The rate of return to pre-injury level of sports in athletes has been shown to be 68.4% within 2 years following revision ACL. Data from the Norwegian registry revealed the cumulative estimated proportion of patients undergoing a re-revision ACLR at 1-, 2-, 5-, and 8-years following revision ACLR to be 0.4, 3.0, 6.5, and 9.0% respectively [187]. Factors associated with less satisfactory results of revision ACL compared to primary ACLR are not yet fully elucidated. Concomitant cartilage and meniscal pathology are thought to be contributing factors to inferior outcomes following revision ACLR compared to primary ACLR [181, 203]. Chronic postoperative pain is thought to be one of the most significant complications following revision ACLR. However, as patients with significant pain typically refrain from further surgery, incidence and implications of chronic pain as a complication of revision ACLR are not well elucidated. Other complications include infection, residual instability, graft re-rupture, arthrofibrosis, DVT as well as CRPS.

## References

1. Akhtar MA, Bhattacharya R & Keating JF. Generalised ligamentous laxity and revision ACL surgery: is there a relation? Knee. 2016;23:1148–1153. https://doi.org/10.1016/j.knee.2015.11.006.
2. Akoto R, Alm L, Drenck TC, Frings J, Krause M, Frosch KH. Slope-correction osteotomy with lateral extra-articular tenodesis and revision anterior cruciate ligament reconstruction is highly effective in treating high-grade anterior knee laxity. Am J Sports Med. 2020;48:3478–85. https://doi.org/10.1177/0363546520966327.
3. Alm L, Krause M, Frosch KH, Akoto R. Preoperative medial knee instability is an underestimated risk factor for failure of revision ACL reconstruction. Knee Surg Sports Traumatol Arthrosc. 2020;28:2458–67. https://doi.org/10.1007/s00167-020-06133-y.
4. Alomar AZ, Alfayez SM, Somily AM. Hamstring autografts are associated with a high rate of contamination in anterior cruciate ligament reconstruction. Knee Surg Sports Traumatol Arthrosc. 2018;26:1357–61. https://doi.org/10.1007/s00167-017-4686-4.
5. Baer GS, Harner CD. Clinical outcomes of allograft versus autograft in anterior cruciate ligament reconstruction. Clin Sports Med. 2007;26:661–681. https://doi.org/10.1016/j.csm.2007.06.010.
6. Barber-Westin S, Noyes FR. One in 5 athletes sustain reinjury upon return to high-risk sports after ACL reconstruction: a systematic review in 1239 athletes younger than 20 years. Sports Health. 2020;12:587–97. https://doi.org/10.1177/1941738120912846.
7. Barié A, Ehmann Y, Jaber A, Huber J, Streich NA. Revision ACL reconstruction using quadriceps or hamstring autografts leads to similar results after 4 years: good objective stability but low rate of return to pre-injury sport level. Knee Surg Sports Traumatol Arthrosc. 2019;27:3527–35. https://doi.org/10.1007/s00167-019-05444-z.
8. Bedi A, Warren RF, Wojtys EM, Oh YK, Ashton-Miller JA, Oltean H, Kelly BT. Restriction in hip internal rotation is associated with an increased risk of ACL injury. Knee Surg Sports Traumatol Arthrosc. 2016;24:2024–2031. https://doi.org/10.1007/s00167-014-3299-4. Downloaded from Bioscientwiwfiwca.e.cfomrtoatpe0n5/r1e0v/i2e0w23s.o01rg:05:53PM via free access.
9. Belk JW, Littlefield CP, Smith JH, McCulloch PC, McCarty EC, Frank RM, Kraeutler MJ. Autograft demonstrates superior outcomes for revision anterior cruciate ligament reconstruction when compared with allograft: a systematic review. Am J Sports Med. 2023;52:859–867.https://doi.org/10.1177/03635465231152232.

10. Bernhardson AS, Aman ZS, Dornan GJ, Kemler BR, Storaci HW, Brady AW, Nakama GY & LaPrade RF. Tibial slope and its effect on force in anterior cruciate ligament grafts: anterior cruciate ligament force increases linearly as posterior tibial slope increases. Am J Sports Med. 2019;47:296–302. https://doi.org/10.1177/0363546518820302.
11. Beynnon BD, Uh BS, Johnson RJ, Fleming BC, Renstrom PA, Nichols CE. The elongation behavior of the anterior cruciate ligament graft in vivo. A long-term follow-up study. Am J Sports Med. 2001;29(2):161–166.
12. Biau DJ, Tournoux C, Katsahian S, Schranz PJ, Nizard RS. Bone-patellar tendon-bone autografts versus hamstring autografts for reconstruction of anterior cruciate ligament: meta-analysis. BMJ. 2006;332:995–1001. https://doi.org/10.1136/bmj.38784.384109.2F.
13. Bouguennec N, Odri GA, Graveleau N, Colombet P. Comparative reproducibility of TELOSTM and GNRB® for instrumental measurement of anterior tibial translation in normal knees. Orthop Traumatol Surg Res. 2015;101:301–5. https://doi.org/10.1016/j.otsr.2015.01.007.
14. Brophy RH, Haas AK, Huston LJ, Nwosu SK, MARS Group, Wright RW. Association of meniscal status, lower extremity alignment, and body mass index with chondrosis at revision anterior cruciate ligament reconstruction. Am J Sports Med. 2015;43:1616–1622. https://doi.org/10.1177/0363546515578838.
15. Bumberger A, Koller U, Hofbauer M, Tiefenboeck TM, Hajdu S, Windhager R, Waldstein W. Ramp lesions are frequently missed in ACL-deficient knees and should be repaired in case of instability. Knee Surg Sports Traumatol Arthrosc. 2020;28:840–54. https://doi.org/10.1007/s00167-019-05521-3.
16. Burnham JM, Wright V. Update on Anterior Cruciate Ligament Rupture and Care in the Female Athlete. Clin Sports Med. 2017 Oct;36(4):703–15. https://doi.org/10.1016/j.csm.2017.05.004. PMID: 28886823.
17. Carson EW, Anisko EM, Restrepo C, Panariello RA, O'Brien SJ, Warren RF. Revision anterior 402 cruciate ligament reconstruction: etiology of failures and clinical results. J Knee Surg. 2004;17(3):127–32.
18. Chen Y, Chua KHZ, Singh A, Tan JH, Chen X, Tan SH, Tai BC, Lingaraj K. Outcome of single-bundle hamstring anterior cruciate ligament reconstruction using the anteromedial versus the transtibial technique: a systematic review and meta-analysis. Arthroscopy. 2015;31:1784–94. https://doi.org/10.1016/j.arthro.2015.06.001.
19. Chen H, Tie K, Qi Y, Li B, Chen B, Chen L. Anteromedial versus transtibial technique in single-bundle autologous hamstring ACL reconstruction: a meta-analysis of prospective randomized controlled trials. J Orthopaed Surg Res. 2017;12:167. https://doi.org/10.1186/s13018-017-0671-3.
20. Chen JL, Allen CR, Stephens TE, Haas AK, Huston LJ, Wright RW, Feeley BT, Multicenter ACL Revision Study (MARS) Group. Differences in mechanisms of failure, intraoperative findings, and surgical characteristics between single- and multiple- revision ACL reconstructions: a MARS cohort study. Am J Sports Med. 2013;41:1571–1578. https://doi.org/10.1177/0363546513487980.
21. Ciccotti MC, Secrist E, Tjoumakaris F, Ciccotti MG, Freedman KB. Anatomic anterior cruciate ligament reconstruction via independent tunnel drilling: a systematic review of randomized controlled trials comparing patellar tendon and hamstring autografts. Arthroscopy. 2017;33:1062-1071.e5. https://doi.org/10.1016/j.arthro.2017.01.033.
22. Clatworthy MG, Annear P, Bulow JU, Bartlett RJ. Tunnel widening in anterior cruciate ligament reconstruction: a prospective evaluation of hamstring and patella tendon grafts. Knee Surg Sports Traumatol Arthrosc. 1999;7(3):138–45.
23. Cohen D, Yao PF, Uddandam A, de Sa D, Arakgi ME. Etiology of Failed Anterior Cruciate Ligament Reconstruction: a Scoping Review. Curr Rev Musculoskelet Med. 2022 Oct;15(5):394–401. https://doi.org/10.1007/s12178-022-09776-1. Epub 2022 Jul 19. PMID: 35852699; PMCID: PMC9463419.
24. Colatruglio M, Flanigan DC, Long J, DiBartola AC & Magnussen RA. Outcomes of 1-versus 2-stage revision anterior cruciate ligament reconstruction: a systematic review and

meta-analysis. Am J o Sports Med. 2021;49:798–804. https://doi.org/10.1177/0363546520923090.

25. Condello V, Zdanowicz U, Di Matteo B, Spalding T, Gelber PE, Adravanti P, Heuberer P, Dimmen S, Sonnery-Cottet B, Hulet C, Bonomo M, Kon E. Allograft tendons are a safe and effective option for revision ACL reconstruction: a clinical review. Knee Surg Sports Traumatol Arthrosc. 2019 Jun;27(6):1771–81. https://doi.org/10.1007/s00167-018-5147-4. Epub 2018 Sep 21. PMID: 30242455.
26. Costa GG, Grassi A, Lo Presti M, Cialdella S, Zamparini E, Viale P, Filardo G, Zaffagnini S. White blood cell count is the most reliable test for the diagnosis of septic arthritis after anterior cruciate ligament reconstruction: an observational study of 38 patients. Arthroscopy. 2021;37:1522-1530.e2. https://doi.org/10.1016/j.arthro.2020.11.047.
27. Costa GG, Grassi A, Perelli S, Agrò G, Bozzi F, Lo Presti M, Zaffagnini S. Age over 50 years is not a contraindication for anterior cruciate ligament reconstruction. Knee Surg Sports Traumatol Arthrosc. 2019;27:3679–91. https://doi.org/10.1007/s00167-019-05450-1.
28. Cristiani R, van de Bunt F, Kvist J, Stålman A. High prevalence of meniscal ramp lesions in anterior cruciate ligament injuries. Knee Surg Sports Traumatol Arthrosc. 2023;31:316–24. https://doi.org/10.1007/s00167-022-07135-8.
29. Cristiani R, Engström B, Edman G, Forssblad M, Stålman A. Revision anterior cruciate ligament reconstruction restores knee laxity but shows inferior functional knee outcome compared with primary reconstruction. Knee Surg Sports Traumatol Arthrosc. 2019 Jan;27(1):137–45. https://doi.org/10.1007/s00167-018-5059-3. Epub 2018 Jul 17. PMID: 30014185; PMCID: PMC6510814.
30. Crum R, Darren de SA, Ayeni OR, Musahl V. No difference between extraction drilling and serial dilation for tibial tunnel preparation in anterior cruciate ligament reconstruction: a systematic review. J ISAKOS Joint Disorders Orthopaed Sports Med 2018;3. https://doi.org/10.1136/jisakos-2017-000191.
31. DePhillipo NN, Dekker TJ, Aman ZS, Bernholt D, Grantham WJ, LaPrade RF. Incidence and healing rates of meniscal tears in patients undergoing repair during the first stage of 2-stage revision anterior cruciate ligament reconstruction. Am J Sports Med. 2019;47:3389–3395. https://doi.org/10.1177/0363546519878421.
32. DePhillipo NN, Moatshe G, Chahla J, Aman ZS, Storaci HW, Morris ER, Robbins CM, Engebretsen L, LaPrade RF. Quantitative and qualitative assessment of the posterior medial meniscus anatomy: defining meniscal ramp lesions. Am J Sports Med. 2019;47:372–378. https://doi.org/10.1177/0363546518814258.
33. Dejour D, Saffarini M, Demey G, Baverel L. Tibial slope correction combined with second revision ACL produces good knee stability and prevents graft rupture. Knee Surg Sports Traumatol Arthrosc. 2015;23:2846–52. https://doi.org/10.1007/s00167-015-3758-6.
34. Dejour D, Pungitore M, Valluy J, Nover L, Saffarini M, Demey G. Preoperative laxity in ACL-deficient knees increases with posterior tibial slope and medial meniscal tears. Knee Surg Sports Traumatol Arthrosc. 2019;27:564–572. https://doi.org/10.1007/s00167-018-5180-3.
35. Dekker TJ, Godin JA, Dale KM, Garrett WE, Taylor DC, Riboh JC. Return to sport after pediatric anterior cruciate ligament reconstruction and its effect on subsequent anterior cruciate ligament injury. J Bone Joint Surg Am. 2017;99:897–904. https://doi.org/10.2106/JBJS.16.00758.
36. Denti M, Lo Vetere D, Bait C, Schonhuber H, Melegati G, Volpi P. Revision anterior cruciate ligament reconstruction: causes of failure, surgical technique, and clinical results. Am J Sports Med. 2008;36(10):1896–902.
37. Diquattro E, Jahnke S, Traina F, Perdisa F, Becker R, Kopf S. ACL surgery: reasons for failure and management. EFORT Open Rev. 2023 May 9;8(5):319–30. https://doi.org/10.1530/EOR-23-0085. PMID: 37158438; PMCID: PMC10233814.
38. Dragoo JL, Kalisvaart M, Smith KM, Pappas G, Golish R. Single-stage revision anterior cruciate ligament reconstruction using bone grafting for posterior or widening tibial tunnels restores stability of the knee and improves clinical outcomes. Knee Surg Sports Traumatol Arthrosc. 2019 Nov;27(11):3713–21. https://doi.org/10.1007/s00167-019-05467-6. Epub 2019 Apr 12. PMID: 30980118.

39. Eberhardt C, Kurth AH, Hailer N, Jager A. Revision ACL reconstruction using autogenous patellar tendon graft. Knee Surg Sports Traumatol Arthrosc. 2000;8(5):290–5.
40. Engebretsen L, Benum P, Fasting O, Mølster A & Strand T. A prospective, randomized study of three surgical techniques for treatment of acute ruptures of the anterior cruciate ligament. Am J Sports Med. 1990;18:585–590. https://doi.org/10.1177/036354659001800605.
41. Engler ID, Sylvia SM, Salzler MJ, Forlizzi JM, Gill IV TJ. Single-stage revision anterior cruciate ligament reconstruction using the stacked screws technique. Arthroscopy Techniques. 2022;11(7):e1341–5. ISSN 2212-6287. https://doi.org/10.1016/j.eats.2022.03.020.
42. Erickson BJ, Cvetanovich G, Waliullah K, Khair M, Smith P, Bach B, Sherman S. Two-stage revision anterior cruciate ligament reconstruction. Orthopedics. 2016;39:e456–64. https://doi.org/10.3928/01477447-20160324-01.
43. Erickson BJ, Cvetanovich GL, Frank RM, Riff AJ & Bach BRJ. Revision ACL reconstruction: a critical analysis review. JBJS Rev. 2017;5:e1. https://doi.org/10.2106/JBJS.RVW.16.00094.
44. Ernat JJ, Rakowski DR, Millett PJ. Single-Stage Anterior Cruciate Ligament Revision Reconstruction Using an Allograft Bone Dowel for a Malpositioned and Widened Femoral Tunnel. Arthrosc Tech. 2021 Jun 20;10(7):e1793–97. https://doi.org/10.1016/j.eats.2021.03.023. PMID: 34336577; PMCID: PMC8322569.
45. Espregueira-Mendes J, Pereira H, Monteiro A, Oliveira J, Reis Rui L, Ripóll P, Thomas N. ACL Two-Stage Revision Surgery: practical guide. 2014. https://doi.org/10.1007/978-3-642-45349-6_36
46. Fahey M, Indelicato PA (1994) Bone tunnel enlargement after anterior cruciate ligament replacement. Am J Sports Med 22(3):410–414; 18(11):1573–1575
47. Ferretti A, Monaco E, Caperna L, Palma T, Conteduca F. Revision ACL reconstruction using contralateral hamstrings. Knee Surg Sports Traumatol Arthrosc. 2013;21:690–5. https://doi.org/10.1007/s00167-012-2039-x.
48. Ferretti A, Monaco E, Labianca L, De Carli A, Conteduca F. Double bundle or single bundle plus extra-articular tenodesis in ACL reconstruction? A CAOS study. Knee Surg Sports Traumatol Arthrosc. 2008;16(1):98.
49. Feucht MJ, Grande E, Brunhuber J, Rosenstiel N, Burgkart R, Imhoff AB, Braun S. Biomechanical evaluation of different suture materials for arthroscopic transtibial pull-out repair of posterior meniscus root tears. Knee Surg Sports Traumatol Arthrosc. 2015;23:132–9. https://doi.org/10.1007/s00167-013-2656-z.
50. Feucht MJ, Mauro CS, Brucker PU, Imhoff AB, Hinterwimmer S. The role of the tibial slope in sustaining and treating anterior cruciate ligament injuries. Knee Surg Sports Traumatol Arthrosc. 2013;21:134–45. https://doi.org/10.1007/s00167-012-1941-6.
51. Fox JA, Pierce M, Bojchuk J, Hayden J, Bush-Joseph CA, Bach BR Jr. Revision anterior cruciate ligament reconstruction with nonirradiated freshfrozen patellar tendon allograft. Arthroscopy. 2004;20(8):787–94.
52. Franceschi F, Papalia R, Del Buono A, Zampogna B, Diaz Balzani L, Maffulli N, Denaro V. Two-stage procedure in anterior cruciate ligament revision surgery: a five-year follow-up prospective study. Int Orthop. 2013;37:1369–74. https://doi.org/10.1007/s00264-013-1886-5.
53. Fules PJ, Madhav RT, Goddard RK, Mowbray MA. Revision anterior cruciate ligament reconstruction using autografts with a polyester fi xation device. Knee. 2003;10(4):335–40.
54. Garofalo R, Djahangiri A, Siegrist O. Revision anterior cruciate ligament reconstruction with quadriceps tendon-patellar bone autograft. Arthroscopy. 2006;22(2):205–14.
55. George MS, Dunn WR, Spindler KP. Current concepts review: revision anterior cruciate ligament reconstruction. Am J Sports Med. 2006;34(12):2026–37.
56. George MS, Dunn WR, Spindler KP. Current concepts review: revision anterior cruciate ligament reconstruction. Am J Sports Med. 2006 Dec;34(12):2026–37. https://doi.org/10.1177/0363546506295026. Epub 2006 Nov 7. PMID: 17092921.
57. Getelman MH, Friedman MJ. Revision anterior cruciate ligament reconstruction surgery. J Am Acad Orthop Surg. 1999;7(3):189–98.
58. Getgood A, Brown C, Lording T, Amis A, Claes S, Geeslin A, Musahl V, ALC Consensus Group. The anterolateral complex of the knee: results from the International ALC Consensus

Group Meeting. Knee Surg Sports Traumatol Arthrosc. 2019;27:166–176. https://doi.org/10.1007/s00167-018-5072-6.

59. Getgood AMJ, Bryant DM, Litchfield R, Heard M, McCormack RG, Rezansoff A, Peterson D, Bardana D, MacDonald PB, Verdonk PCM, et al. Lateral extra-articular tenodesis reduces failure of hamstring tendon autograft anterior cruciate ligament reconstruction: 2-year outcomes from the STABILITY study randomized clinical trial. Am J Sports Med. 2020; 48:285–297. https://doi.org/10.1177/0363546519896333.
60. Gifstad T, Drogset JO, Viset A, Grontvedt T, Hortemo GS. Inferior results after revision ACL reconstructions: a comparison with primary ACL reconstructions. Knee Surg Sports Traumatol Arthrosc. 2013;21(9):2011–8.
61. Gifstad T, Drogset JO, Viset A, Grøntvedt T, Hortemo GS. Inferior results after revision ACL reconstructions: a comparison with primary ACL reconstructions. Knee Surg Sports Traumatol Arthrosc. 2013;21:2011–8. https://doi.org/10.1007/s00167-012-2336-4.
62. Goertzen MJ, Buitkamp J, Clahsen H, Mollmann M. Cell survival following bone-anterior cruciate ligament-bone allograft transplantation: DNA fi ngerprints, segregation, and collagen morphological analysis of multiple markers in the canine model. Arch Orthop Trauma Surg. 1998;117(4–5):208–14.
63. Gracia G, Cavaignac M, Marot V, Mouarbes D, Laumonerie P, Cavaignac E. Epidemiology of combined injuries of the secondary stabilizers in ACL-deficient knees: medial meniscal ramp lesion, lateral meniscus root tear, and ALL tear: a prospective case series of 602 patients with ACL tears from the SANTI study group. Am J Sports Med. 2022;50:1843–9. https://doi.org/10.1177/03635465221092767.
64. Granan LP, Forssblad M, Lind M, Engebretsen L. The Scandinavian ACL registries 2004–2007: baseline epidemiology. Acta Orthop. 2009;80(5):563–7.
65. Grassi A, Bailey JR, Signorelli C, Carbone G, Tchonang Wakam A, Lucidi GA, Zaffagnini S. Magnetic resonance imaging after anterior cruciate ligament reconstruction: a practical guide. World J Orthoped. 2016;7:638–649. https://doi.org/10.5312/wjo.v7.i10.638.
66. Grassi A, Zicaro JP, Costa-Paz M, Samuelsson K, Wilson A, Zaffagnini S, Condello V, ESSKA Arthroscopy Committee. Good mid-term outcomes and low rates of residual rotatory laxity, complications and failures after revision anterior cruciate ligament reconstruction (ACL) and lateral extra-articular tenodesis (LET). Knee Surg Sports Traumatol Arthrosc. 2020;28:418–431. https://doi.org/10.1007/s00167-019-05625-w.
67. Grossman MG, ElAttrache NS, Shields CL, Glousman RE. Revision anterior cruciate ligament reconstruction: three- to nine-year follow-up. Arthroscopy. 2005;21(4):418–23.
68. Guimarães TM, Giglio PN, Sobrado MF, Bonadio MB, Gobbi RG, Pécora JR & Helito CP. Knee hyperextension greater than 5° is a risk factor for failure in ACL reconstruction using hamstring graft. Orthopaed J Sports Med. 2021;9:23259671211056325. https://doi.org/10.1177/23259671211056325.
69. Gupta A, Tejpal T, Shanmugaraj A, Horner NS, Simunovic N, Duong A, Ayeni OR. Surgical techniques, outcomes, indications, and complications of simultaneous high tibial osteotomy and anterior cruciate ligament revision surgery: a systematic review. HSS J. 2019;15:176–84. https://doi.org/10.1007/s11420-018-9630-8.
70. Hemmerich A, van der Merwe W, Vaughan CL. Measuring three-dimensional knee kinematics under torsional loading. J Biomech. 2009;42:183–6. https://doi.org/10.1016/j.jbiomech.2008.10.021.
71. Hettrich CM, Dunn WR, Reinke EK, MOON Group, Spindler KP. The rate of subsequent surgery and predictors after anterior cruciate ligament reconstruction: two- and 6-year follow-up results from a multicenter cohort. Am J Sports Med. 2013;41:1534–1540. https://doi.org/10.1177/0363546513490277.
72. Hoher J, Moller HD, Fu FH. Bone tunnel enlargement after anterior cruciate ligament reconstruction: fact or fi ction? Knee Surg Sports Traumatol Arthrosc. 1998;6(4):231–40.
73. Hoshino Y, Araujo P, Irrgang JJ, Fu FH, Musahl V. An image analysis method to quantify the lateral pivot shift test. Knee Surg Sports Traumatol Arthrosc. 2012;20:703–7. https://doi.org/10.1007/s00167-011-1845-x.

74. Hoshino Y, Kuroda R, Nagamune K, Yagi M, Mizuno K, Yamaguchi M, Muratsu H, Yoshiya S, Kurosaka M. In vivo measurement of the pivot-shift test in the anterior cruciate ligament-deficient knee using an electromagnetic device. Am J Sports Med. 2007;35:1098–104. https://doi.org/10.1177/0363546507299447.
75. Hoshino Y, Araujo P, Ahlden M, Moore CG, Kuroda R, Zaffagnini S, Karlsson J, Fu FH, Musahl V. Standardized pivot shift test improves measurement accuracy. Knee Surg Sports Traumatol Arthrosc. 2012;20:732–736. https://doi.org/10.1007/s00167-011-1850-0.
76. hyperextension is a predictor of failure in an anterior cruciate ligament revision cohort: a report from the MARS group. Am J Sports Med. 2018;46:2836–41. https://doi.org/10.1177/0363546518777732.
77. Häner M, Bierke S, Petersen W. Anterior cruciate ligament revision surgery: ipsilateral quadriceps versus contralateral semitendinosus-gracilis autografts. Arthroscopy. 2016;32:2308–17. https://doi.org/10.1016/j.arthro.2016.03.020.
78. Imhoff FB, Mehl J, Comer BJ, Obopilwe E, Cote MP, Feucht MJ, Wylie JD, Imhoff AB, Arciero RA, Beitzel K. Slope-reducing tibial osteotomy decreases ACL-graft forces and anterior tibial translation under axial load. Knee Surg Sports Traumatol Arthrosc. 2019;27:3381–9. https://doi.org/10.1007/s00167-019-05360-2.
79. Johnson DL, Swenson TM, Irrgang JJ, Fu FH, Harner CD. Revision anterior cruciate ligament surgery: experience from Pittsburgh. Clin Orthop Relat Res. 1996;325:100–9.
80. Kaeding CC, Aros B, Pedroza A, Pifel E, Amendola A, Andrish JT, Dunn WR, Marx RG, McCarty EC, Parker RD, et al. Allograft versus autograft anterior cruciate ligament reconstruction: predictors of failure from a MOON prospective longitudinal cohort. Sports Health. 2011;3:73–81. https://doi.org/10.1177/1941738110386185.
81. Kamath GV, Redfern JC, Greis PE, Burks RT. Revision anterior cruciate ligament reconstruction. Am J Sports Med. 2011;39:199–217. https://doi.org/10.1177/0363546510370929.
82. Kanakamedala AC, Edgar CM, Fanelli GC, Musahl V, Alaia MJ. Surgical considerations in revision anterior cruciate ligament reconstruction. Instruct Course Lect. 2022;71:475–87.
83. Kartus J, Movin T, Karlsson J. Donor-site morbidity and anterior knee problems after anterior cruciate ligament reconstruction using autografts. Arthroscopy. 2001;17(9):971–80.
84. Keizer MNJ, Hoogeslag RAG, van Raay JJAM, Otten E, Brouwer RW. Superior return to sports rate after patellar tendon autograft over patellar tendon allograft in revision anterior cruciate ligament reconstruction. Knee Surg Sports Traumatol Arthrosc. 2018 Feb;26(2):574–81. https://doi.org/10.1007/s00167-017-4612-9. Epub 2017 Jun 17. PMID: 28624854.
85. Kim SJ, Park KH, Kim SH, Kim SG, Chun YM. Anterior cruciate ligament reconstruction improves activity-induced pain in comparison with pain at rest in middle- aged patients with significant cartilage degeneration. Am J Sports Med. 2010;38:1343–8. https://doi.org/10.1177/0363546509360406.
86. Kim HS, Seon JK, Jo AR. Current trends in anterior cruciate ligament reconstruction. Knee Surg Relat Res. 2013;25:165–73. https://doi.org/10.5792/ksrr.2013.25.4.165.
87. Kim DH, Bae KC, Kim DW et al. Two-stage revision anterior cruciate ligament reconstruction. Knee Surg & Relat Res 2019;31:10. https://doi.org/10.1186/s43019-019-0010-6
88. Kopf S, Kauert R, Halfpaap J, Jung T, Becker R. A new quantitative method for pivot shift grading. Knee Surg Sports Traumatol Arthrosc. 2012;20:718–23. https://doi.org/10.1007/s00167-012-1903-z.
89. Kosy JD, Mandalia VI. Plain radiographs can be used for routine assessment of ACL reconstruction tunnel position with three-dimensional imaging reserved for research and revision surgery. Knee Surg Sports Traumatol Arthrosc. 2018;26:534–49. https://doi.org/10.1007/s00167-017-4462-5.
90. Kraeutler MJ, Bravman JT, McCarty EC. Bone-patellar tendon-bone autograft versus allograft in outcomes of anterior cruciate ligament reconstruction: a meta-analysis of 5182 patients. Am J Sports Med. 2013 Oct;41(10):2439–48. https://doi.org/10.1177/0363546513484127. Epub 2013 Apr 12. PMID: 23585484.
91. LaPrade RF, Geeslin AG, Chahla J, Cohen M, Engebretsen L, Faucett SC, Getgood AM, Inderhaug E, Johnson DL, Kopf S, et al. Posterior lateral meniscal root and oblique radial tears: the

biomechanical evidence supports repair of these tears, although long-term clinical studies are necessary. Arthroscopy. 2022;38:3095–3101. https://doi.org/10.1016/j.arthro.2022.09.015.

92. Laprade RF, Bernhardson AS, Griffi th CJ, Macalena JA, Wijdicks CA. Correlation of valgus stress radiographs with medial knee ligament injuries: an in vitro biomechanical study. Am J Sports Med. 2010;38(2):330–338.
93. Lee MC, Seong SC, Lee S, Chang CB, Park YK, Jo H, Kim CH. Vertical femoral tunnel placement results in rotational knee laxity after anterior cruciate ligament reconstruction. Arthroscopy. 2007 Jul;23(7):771–8. https://doi.org/10.1016/j.arthro.2007.04.016. PMID: 17637414.
94. Lefevre N, Klouche S, Mirouse G, Herman S, Gerometta A, Bohu Y. Return to sport after primary and revision anterior cruciate ligament reconstruction: a prospective comparative study of 552 patients from the FAST cohort. Am J Sports Med. 2017;45:34–41. https://doi.org/10.1177/0363546516660075.
95. Legnani C, Peretti G, Borgo E, Zini S, Ventura A. Revision anterior cruciate ligament reconstruction with ipsi- or contralateral hamstring tendon grafts. Eur J Orthopaed Surg Traumatol Orthopedie Traumatologie. 2017;27:533–7. https://doi.org/10.1007/s00590-016-1894-4.
96. Li X, Yan L, Li D, Fan Z, Liu H, Wang G, Jiu J, Yang Z, Li JJ, Wang B. Failure modes after anterior cruciate ligament reconstruction: a systematic review and meta- analysis. Int Orthop. 2023;47:719–34. https://doi.org/10.1007/s00264-023-05687-z.
97. Liu X, Zhang H, Feng H, Hong L, Wang XS, Song GY. Is it necessary to repair stable ramp lesions of the medial meniscus during anterior cruciate ligament reconstruction? A prospective randomized controlled trial. Am J Sports Med. 2017;45:1004–11. https://doi.org/10.1177/0363546516682493.
98. Liukkonen R, Ponkilainen V, Reito A. Revision Rates After Primary ACL Reconstruction Performed Between 1969 and 2018: A Systematic Review and Metaregression Analysis. The Orthopaedic Journal of Sports Medicine 2022;10. https://doi.org/10.1177/23259671221110191.
99. Liukkonen RJ, Ponkilainen VT & Reito A. Revision rates after primary ACL reconstruction performed between 1969 and 2018: A systematic review and metaregression analysis. Orthopaed J Sports Med. 2022;10:23259671221110191. https://doi.org/10.1177/23259671221110191.
100. Lopomo N, Zaffagnini S, Bignozzi S, Visani A, Marcacci M. Pivot-shift test: analysis and quantification of knee laxity parameters using a navigation system. J Orthop Res. 2010;28:164–9. https://doi.org/10.1002/jor.20966.
101. Lorbach O, Kieb M, Herbort M, Weyers I, Raschke M, Engelhardt M. The influence of the medial meniscus in different conditions on anterior tibial translation in the anterior cruciate deficient knee. Int Orthopaed. 2015;39:681–687. https://doi.org/10.1007/s00264-014-2581-x.
102. Lubowitz JH, Bernardini BJ, Reid JB 3rd. Current concepts review: comprehensive physical examination for instability of the knee. Am J Sports Med. 2008;36(3):577–94.
103. Lynch TS, Parker RD, Patel RM, Andrish JT, MOON Group, Spindler KP, Amendola A, Brophy RH, Dunn WR, Flanigan DC, et al. The impact of the Multicenter Orthopaedic Outcomes Network (MOON) research on anterior cruciate ligament reconstruction and orthopaedic practice. J Am Acad Orthopaed Surg. 2015:23;154–163. https://doi.org/10.5435/JAAOS-D-14-00005.
104. L'Insalata JC, Klatt B, Fu FH, Harner CD. Tunnel expansion following anterior cruciate ligamen reconstruction: a comparison of hamstring and patellar tendon autografts. Knee Surg Sports Traumatol Arthrosc. 1997;5(4):234–8.
105. MARS Group, Huston L, Haas A. Factors influencing graft choice in revision anterior cruciate ligament reconstruction in the MARS Group. J Knee Surg. 2016;29:458–463. https://doi.org/10.1055/s-0035-1564723.
106. MARS Group, Wright RW, Huston LJ, Haas AK, Pennings JS, Allen CR, Cooper DE, DeBerardino TM, Dunn WR, Lantz BBA, et al. Association between graft choice and 6-year outcomes of revision anterior cruciate ligament reconstruction in the MARS cohort. Am J Sports Med. 2021;49:2589–2598. https://doi.org/10.1177/03635465211027170.

107. MARS Group, Wright RW, Huston LJ, Spindler KP, Dunn WR, Haas AK, Allen CR, Cooper DE, DeBerardino TM, Lantz BB, et al. Descriptive epidemiology of the Multicenter ACL Revision Study (MARS) cohort. Am J Sports Med. 2010;38:1979–1986. https://doi.org/10.1177/0363546510378645. www.efortopenreviews.org.
108. MARS Group & MARS Group. Effect of graft choice on the outcome of revision anterior cruciate ligament reconstruction in the Multicenter ACL Revision Study (MARS) Cohort. Am J Sports Med. 2014;42:2301–2310. https://doi.org/10.1177/0363546514549005.
109. MARS Group, Cooper DE, Dunn WR, Huston LJ, Haas AK, Spindler KP, Allen CR, Anderson AF, DeBerardino TM, Lantz BBA, et al. Physiologic preoperative knee
110. MOON Knee Group, Spindler KP, Huston LJ, Zajichek A, Reinke EK, Amendola A, Andrish JT, Brophy RH, Dunn WR, Flanigan DC, et al. Anterior cruciate ligament reconstruction in high school and college-aged athletes: does autograft choice influence anterior cruciate ligament revision rates? Am J Sports Med. 2020;48:298–309. https://doi.org/10.1177/0363546519892991.
111. Machotka Z, Scarborough I, Duncan W, Kumar S, Perraton L. Anterior cruciate ligament repair with LARS (ligament advanced reinforcement system): a systematic review. Sports Med Arthrosc Rehabil Ther Technol. 2010;2(29):403.
112. Magnussen RA, Lawrence JTR, West RL, Toth AP, Taylor DC & Garrett WE. Graft size and patient age are predictors of early revision after anterior cruciate ligament reconstruction with hamstring autograft. Arthroscopy. 2012;28:526–531. https://doi.org/10.1016/j.arthro.2011.11.024.
113. Makhmalbaf H, Moradi A, Ganji S, Omidi-Kashani F. Accuracy of Lachman and anterior drawer tests for anterior cruciate ligament injuries. Arch Bone Joint Surg. 2013;1:94–7.
114. Malinin TI, Levitt RL, Bashore C, Temple HT, Mnaymneh W. A study of retrieved allografts used to replace anterior cruciate ligaments. Arthroscopy. 2002;18(2):163–70.
115. Marchant MHJ, Willimon SC, Vinson E, Pietrobon R, Garrett WE, Higgins LD. Comparison of plain radiography, computed tomography, and magnetic resonance imaging in the evaluation of bone tunnel widening after anterior cruciate ligament reconstruction. Knee Surg Sports Traumatol Arthrosc. 2010;18:1059–64. https://doi.org/10.1007/s00167-009-0952-4.
116. Mariscalco MW, Flanigan DC, Mitchell J, Pedroza AD, Jones MH, Andrish JT, Parker RD, Kaeding CC, Magnussen RA. The influence of hamstring autograft size on patient-reported outcomes and risk of revision after anterior cruciate ligament reconstruction: a Multicenter Orthopaedic Outcomes Network (MOON) Cohort Study. Arthroscopy. 2013;29:1948–53. https://doi.org/10.1016/j.arthro.2013.08.025.
117. Marrale J, Morrissey MC, Haddad FS. A literature review of autograft and allograft anterior cruciate ligament reconstruction. Knee Surg Sports Traumatol Arthrosc. 2007;15(6):690–704.
118. Martin RK, Wastvedt S, Pareek A, Persson A, Visnes H, Fenstad AM, Moatshe G, Wolfson J, Lind M, Engebretsen L. Machine learning algorithm to predict anterior cruciate ligament revision demonstrates external validity. Knee Surg Sports Traumatol Arthrosc 2022;30:368–75. https://doi.org/10.1007/s00167-021-06828-w
119. Martinek V, Friederich NF. Tibial and pretibial cyst formation after anterior cruciate ligament reconstruction with bioabsorbable interference screw fi xation. Arthroscopy. 1999;15(3):317–20.
120. Mascarenhas R. Editorial commentary: osseous anatomy of the knee in female patients is a significant risk factor for anterior cruciate ligament injury and anterior cruciate ligament graft failure. Arthroscopy. 2022;38:1605–7. https://doi.org/10.1016/j.arthro.2021.11.042.
121. Matsumoto Y, Takahashi T, Hatayama K, Kubo T, Higuchi H, Kimura M, Takeshita K. Medial meniscal ramp lesion repair concomitant with anterior cruciate ligament reconstruction did not contribute to better anterior knee stability and structural properties after cyclic loading: a porcine model. Arthrosc Sports Med Rehabil. 2021;3:e1967–73. https://doi.org/10.1016/j.asmr.2021.09.019.
122. de Mees TTCR, Reijman M, Waarsing JH, Meuffels DE. Posteriorly positioned femoral grafts decrease long-term failure in anterior cruciate ligament reconstruction, femoral and tibial graft positions did not affect long-term reported outcome. Knee Surg Sports Traumatol Arthrosc. 2022;30:2003–13. https://doi.org/10.1007/s00167-022-06871-1.

123. Mehl J, Otto A, Kia C, Murphy M, Obopilwe E, Imhoff FB, Feucht MJ, Imhoff AB, Arciero RA, Beitzel K. Osseous valgus alignment and posteromedial ligament complex deficiency lead to increased ACL graft forces. Knee Surg Sports Traumatol Arthrosc. 2020;28:1119–29. https://doi.org/10.1007/s00167-019-05770-2.
124. Midttun E, Andersen MT, Engebretsen L, Visnes H, Fenstad AM, Gjertsen JE, Persson A. Good validity in the Norwegian Knee ligament Register: assessment of data quality for key variables in primary and revision cruciate ligament reconstructions from 2004 to 2013. BMC Musculoskeletal Disorders. 2022;23:231. https://doi.org/10.1186/s12891-022-05183-2.
125. Minami T, Muneta T, Sekiya I, Watanabe T, Mochizuki T, Horie M, Katagiri H, Otabe K, Ohara T, Katakura M, et al. Lateral meniscus posterior root tear contributes to anterolateral rotational instability and meniscus extrusion in anterior cruciate ligament-injured patients. Knee Surg Sports Traumatol Arthrosc. 2018;26:1174–81. https://doi.org/10.1007/s00167-017-4569-8.
126. Mitchell JJ, Chahla J, Dean CS, Cinque M, Matheny LM, LaPrade RF. Outcomes after 1-stage versus 2-stage revision anterior cruciate ligament reconstruction. Am J Sports Med. 2017;45:1790–1798. https://doi.org/10.1177/0363546517698684.
127. Mouarbes D, Menetrey J, Marot V, Courtot L, Berard E, Cavaignac E. Anterior cruciate ligament reconstruction: a systematic review and meta-analysis of outcomes for quadriceps tendon autograft versus bone-patellar tendon-bone and hamstring-tendon autografts. Am J Sports Med. 2019;47:3531–40. https://doi.org/10.1177/0363546518825340.
128. Mouzopoulos G, Fotopoulos VC, Tzurbakis M. Septic knee arthritis following ACL reconstruction: a systematic review. Knee Surg Sports Traumatol Arthrosc. 2009;17:1033–42. https://doi.org/10.1007/s00167-009-0793-1.
129. Murgier J, Powell A, Young S, Clatworthy M. Effectiveness of thicker hamstring or patella tendon grafts to reduce graft failure rate in anterior cruciate ligament reconstruction in young patients. Knee Surg Sports Traumatol Arthrosc. 2021;29:725–31. https://doi.org/10.1007/s00167-020-05973-y.
130. Musahl V, Voos J, O'Loughlin PF, Stueber V, Kendoff D, Pearle AD. Mechanized pivot shift test achieves greater accuracy than manual pivot shift test. Knee Surg Sports Traumatol Arthrosc. 2010;18:1208–13. https://doi.org/10.1007/s00167-009-1004-9.
131. Myklebust G, Steffen K. Prevention of ACL injuries: how, when and who? Knee Surg Sports Traumatol Arthrosc. 2009;17(8):857–8.
132. Nakano N, Bartlett J, Khanduja V. Is restricted hip movement a risk factor for anterior cruciate ligament injury? J Orthopaed Surg. 2018;26:2309499018799520. https://doi.org/10.1177/2309499018799520.
133. Nebelung W, Becker R, Merkel M, Ropke M. Bone tunnel enlargement after anterior cruciate ligament reconstruction with semitendinosus tendon using Endobutton fi xation on the femoral side. Arthroscopy. 1998;14(8):810–5.
134. Noyes FR, Barber-Westin SD. Anterior cruciate ligament reconstruction with autogenous patellar tendon graft in patients with articular cartilage damage. Am J Sports Med. 1997;25:626–34. https://doi.org/10.1177/036354659702500507.
135. Noyes FR, Barber-Westin SD, Roberts CS. Use of allografts after failed treatment of rupture of the anterior cruciate ligament. J Bone Joint Surg Am. 1994;76(7):1019–31.
136. Ohly NE, Murray IR, Keating JF. Revision anterior cruciate ligament reconstruction: timing of surgery and the incidence of meniscal tears and degenerative change. J Bone Joint Surg Br. 2007;89(8):1051–4.
137. Pandya NK, Feeley B, Lansdown D, Rubenstein W, Allahabadi S. ACL graft failure in professional athletes compared to the pediatric population. Orthop J Sports Med. 2019;7(3 Suppl):2325967119S00102. https://doi.org/10.1177/2325967119S00102. PMCID: PMC6446390.
138. Parkinson B, Robb C, Thomas M, Thompson P, Spalding T. Factors that predict failure in anatomic single-bundle anterior cruciate ligament reconstruction. Am J Sports Med. 2017;45:1529–1536. https://doi.org/10.1177/0363546517691961.
139. Pinczewski LA, Salmon LJ, Jackson WFM, von Bormann RBP, Haslam PG, Tashiro S. Radiological landmarks for placement of the tunnels in single-bundle reconstruction of the anterior

cruciate ligament. Journal of Bone and Joint Surgery. British Volume 2008 90 172–179. https://doi.org/10.1302/0301-620X.90B2.20104.
140. Poehling-Monaghan KL, Salem H, Ross KE, Secrist E, Ciccotti MC, Tjoumakaris F, Ciccotti MG, Freedman KB. Long-term outcomes in anterior cruciate ligament reconstruction: a systematic review of patellar tendon versus hamstring autografts. Orthopaed J Sports Med. 2017;5:2325967117709735. https://doi.org/10.1177/2325967117709735.
141. Porter MD, Shadbolt B, Pomroy S. The augmentation of revision anterior cruciate ligament reconstruction with modified iliotibial band tenodesis to correct the pivot shift: a computer navigation study. Am J Sports Med. 2018;46:839–45. https://doi.org/10.1177/0363546517750123.
142. Ra HJ, Ha JK, Kim JG. One-stage revision anterior cruciate ligament reconstruction with impacted bone graft after failed primary reconstruction. Orthopedics. 2013;36:860–3. https://doi.org/10.3928/01477447-20131021-07.
143. Rappe M, Horodyski M, Meister K, Indelicato PA. Nonirradiated versus irradiated Achilles allograft: in vivo failure comparison. Am J Sports Med. 2007;35(10):1653–8.
144. von Recum J, Gehm J, Guehring T, Vetter SY, von der Linden P, Grützner PA, Schnetzke M. Autologous bone graft versus silicate-substituted calcium phosphate in the treatment of tunnel defects in 2-stage revision anterior cruciate ligament reconstruction: a prospective, randomized controlled study with a minimum follow-up of 2 years. Arthroscopy. 2020;36:178–85. https://doi.org/10.1016/j.arthro.2019.07.035.
145. Robinson J, Huber C, Jaraj P, Colombet P, Allard M, Meyer P. Reduced bone tunnel enlargement post hamstring ACL reconstruction with poly-L-lactic acid/hydroxyapatite bioabsorbable screws. Knee. 2006;13(2):127–31.
146. Rollier JC, Besse JL, Lerat JL, Moyen B. Anterior cruciate ligament revision: analysis and results from a series of 74 cases. Rev Chir Orthop Reparatrice Appar Mot. 2007;93(4):344–50.
147. Safran MR, Harner CD. Technical considerations of revision anterior cruciate ligament surgery. Clin Orthop Relat Res. 1996;325:50–64.
148. Salem HS, Axibal DP, Wolcott ML, Vidal AF, McCarty EC, Bravman JT, Frank RM. Two-stage revision anterior cruciate ligament reconstruction: a systematic review of bone graft options for tunnel augmentation. Am J Sports Med. 2020;48:767–77. https://doi.org/10.1177/0363546519841583.
149. Salmon LJ, Heath E, Akrawi H, Roe JP, Linklater J, Pinczewski LA. 20- year outcomes of anterior cruciate ligament reconstruction with hamstring tendon autograft: the catastrophic effect of age and posterior tibial slope. Am J Sports Med. 2018;46:531–43. https://doi.org/10.1177/0363546517741497.
150. Samitier G, Marcano AI, Alentorn-Geli E, Cugat R, Farmer KW, Moser MW. Failure of Anterior Cruciate Ligament Reconstruction. Arch Bone Jt Surg. 2015 Oct;3(4):220–40. PMID: 26550585; PMCID: PMC4628627.
151. Santiago P, Del Castillo J, Gilbert M, Robert FL. Anterior cruciate ligament reconstruction failure and revision surgery: current concepts, Journal of ISAKOS 2020;5(6):351–8, ISSN 2059–7754, https://doi.org/10.1136/jisakos-2020-000457.
152. Sauer S, Lind M. Bone tunnel enlargement after ACL reconstruction with hamstring autograft is dependent on original bone tunnel diameter. Surg J (N Y). 2017Jun 19;3(2):e96–100. https://doi.org/10.1055/s-0037-1603950.PMID:28825030;PMCID:PMC5553504.
153. Schlumberger M, Schuster P, Schulz M, Immendörfer M, Mayer P, Bartholomä J, Richter J. Traumatic graft rupture after primary and revision anterior cruciate ligament reconstruction: retrospective analysis of incidence and risk factors in 2915 cases. Knee Surg Sports Traumatol Arthrosc. 2017;25:1535–1541. https://doi.org/10.1007/s00167-015-3699-0.
154. Schmücker M, Haraszuk J, Hölmich P, Barfod KW. Graft failure, revision ACLR, and reoperation rates after ACLR with quadriceps tendon versus hamstring tendon autografts: a registry study with review of 475 patients. Am J Sports Med. 2021;49:2136–43. https://doi.org/10.1177/03635465211015172.
155. Schuster P, Schlumberger M, Mayer P, Eichinger M, Geßlein M, Richter J. Soaking of autografts in vancomycin is highly effective in preventing postoperative septic arthritis

after revision anterior cruciate ligament reconstruction. Knee Surg Sports Traumatol Arthrosc. 2020;28:1154–1158. https://doi.org/10.1007/s00167-019-05820-9. www.efortopenreviews.org.

156. Schwartz HE, Matava MJ, Proch FS, et al. The effect of gamma irradiation on anterior cruciate ligament allograft biomechanical and biochemical properties in the caprine model at time zero and at 6 months after surgery. Am J Sports Med. 2006;34(11):1747–55.
157. Serbin PA, Griffin JW, Bonner KF. Single-Stage Revision Anterior Cruciate Ligament Reconstruction Using Fast-Setting Bone Graft Substitutes. Arthrosc Tech. 2020 Jan 28;9(2):e225–31. https://doi.org/10.1016/j.eats.2019.10.002. PMID: 32099776; PMCID: PMC7029178.
158. Servant C. Editorial Commentary: During Anterior Cruciate Ligament Reconstruction, Lateral Extra-Articular Procedures Have Risks and Should be Reserved for Proper Indications: Do Not LET ALL Revision Anterior Cruciate Ligament Reconstructions Be the Same. Arthroscopy. 2023 Feb;39(2):320–3. https://doi.org/10.1016/j.arthro.2022.08.028. PMID: 36603999.
159. Shekhar A, Tapasvi S, Williams A. Outcomes of combined lateral meniscus posterior root repair and anterior cruciate ligament reconstruction. Orthopaed J Sports Med. 2022;10:23259671221083318. https://doi.org/10.1177/23259671221083318.
160. Shelbourne KD, O'Shea JJ. Revision anterior cruciate ligament reconstruction using the contralateral bone-patellar tendon-bone graft. Instr Course Lect. 2002;51:343–6.
161. Shelbourne KD, Stube KC. Anterior cruciate ligament (ACL)-deficient knee with degenerative arthrosis: treatment with an isolated autogenous patellar tendon ACL reconstruction. Knee Surg Sports Traumatol Arthrosc. 1997;5:150–156. https://doi.org/10.1007/s001670050043.
162. Shelbourne KD, Roberson TA, Gray T. Long-term evaluation of posterior lateral meniscus root tears left in situ at the time of anterior cruciate ligament reconstruction. Am J Sports Med. 2011;39:1439–1443. https://doi.org/10.1177/0363546511398212.
163. Shino K, Inoue M, Horibe S, Nagano J, Ono K. Maturation of allograft tendons transplanted into the knee. An arthroscopic and histological study. J Bone Joint Surg Br. 1988;70(4):556–560.
164. Shino K, Kawasaki T, Hirose H, Gotoh I, Inoue M, Ono K. Replacement of the anterior cruciate ligament by an allogeneic tendon graft. An experimental study in the dog. J Bone Joint Surg Br. 1984; 66(5):672–681
165. Shino K, Oakes BW, Horibe S, Nakata K, Nakamura N. Collagen fi bril populations in human anterior cruciate ligament allografts. Electron microscopic analysis. Am J Sports Med. 1995;23(2):203–208; discussion 209
166. Sonnery-Cottet B, Mogos S, Thaunat M, Archbold P, Fayard JM, Freychet B, Clechet J, Chambat P. Proximal tibial anterior closing wedge osteotomy in repeat revision of anterior cruciate ligament reconstruction. Am J Sports Med. 2014;42:1873–80.
167. Sundemo D, Hamrin Senorski E, Karlsson L, Horvath A, Juul-Kristensen B, Karlsson J, Ayeni OR, Samuelsson K. Generalised joint hypermobility increases ACL injury risk and is associated with inferior outcome after ACL reconstruction: a systematic review. BMJ Open Sport Exercise Med. 2019;5:e000620. https://doi.org/10.1136/bmjsem-2019-000620.
168. Svantesson E, Hamrin Senorski E, Östergaard M, Grassi A, Krupic F, Westin O, Samuelsson K. Graft choice for anterior cruciate ligament reconstruction with a concomitant non-surgically treated medial collateral ligament injury does not influence the risk of revision. Arthroscopy. 2020;36:199–211. https://doi.org/10.1016/j.arthro.2019.07.015.
169. Taggart TF, Kumar A, Bickerstaff DR. Revision anterior cruciate ligament reconstruction: a midterm patient assessment. Knee. 2004;11(1):29–36.
170. Tashiro Y, Okazaki K, Murakami K, Matsubara H, Osaki K, Iwamoto Y, Nakashima Y. Anterolateral rotatory instability in vivo correlates tunnel position after anterior cruciate ligament reconstruction using bone-patellar tendon-bone graft. World Journal of Orthopedics. 2017;8:913–21. https://doi.org/10.5312/wjo.v8.i12.913.
171. Thaunat M, Fayard JM, Guimaraes TM, Jan N, Murphy CG, Sonnery- CB. Classification and surgical repair of ramp lesions of the medial meniscus. Arthrosc Tech. 2016;5:e871–5. https://doi.org/10.1016/j.eats.2016.04.009.

172. Thomas NP, Kankate R, Wandless F, Pandit H. Revision anterior cruciate ligament reconstruction using a 2-stage technique with bone grafting of the tibial tunnel. Am J Sports Med. 2005;33:1701–1709. https://doi.org/10.1177/0363546505276759
173. Thompson R, Hamilton D, Murray I, Lawson G. Notchplasty is associated with decreased risk of anterior cruciate ligament graft revision. Eur J Orthopaed Surg Traumatol Orthopedie Traumatologie. 2022. https://doi.org/10.1007/s00590-022-03305-z.
174. Tischer T, Paul J, Pape D, Hirschmann MT, Imhoff AB, Hinterwimmer S, Feucht MJ. The impact of osseous malalignment and realignment procedures in knee ligament surgery: a systematic review of the clinical evidence. Orthopaed J Sports Med. 2017;5:2325967117697287. https://doi.org/10.1177/2325967117697287.
175. Toanen C, Demey G, Ntagiopoulos PG, Ferrua P, Dejour D. Is there any benefit in anterior cruciate ligament reconstruction in patients older than 60 years? Am J Sports Med. 2017;45:832–837. https://doi.org/10.1177/0363546516678723.
176. Tohyama H, Beynnon BD, Johnson RJ, Renstrom PA, Arms SW. The effect of anterior cruciate ligament graft elongation at the time of implantation on the biomechanical behavior of the graft and knee. Am J Sports Med. 1996;24(5):608–14.
177. Tomihara T, Hashimoto Y, Taniuchi M, Takigami J, Han C, Shimada N. One-stage revision ACL reconstruction after primary ACL double bundle reconstruction: is bone-patella tendon-bone autograft reliable? Knee Surg Sports Traumatol Arthrosc. 2017;25:1653–61. https://doi.org/10.1007/s00167-017-4483-0.
178. Torres-Claramunt R, Gelber P, Pelfort X, Hinarejos P, Leal-Blanquet J, Pérez-Prieto D, Monllau JC. Managing septic arthritis after knee ligament reconstruction. Int Orthop. 2016;40:607–14. https://doi.org/10.1007/s00264-015-2884-6.
179. Torres-Claramunt R, Pelfort X, Erquicia J, Gil-González S, Gelber PE, Puig L, Monllau JC. Knee joint infection after ACL reconstruction: prevalence, management and functional outcomes. Knee Surg Sports Traumatol Arthrosc. 2013;21:2844–9. https://doi.org/10.1007/s00167-012-2264-3.
180. Trojani C, Beaufils P, Burdin G, Bussière C, Chassaing V, Djian P, Dubrana F, Ehkirch FP, Franceschi JP, Hulet C, et al. Revision ACL reconstruction: influence of a lateral tenodesis. Knee Surg Sports Traumatol Arthrosc. 2012;20:1565–70. https://doi.org/10.1007/s00167-011-1765-9.
181. Trojani C, Sbihi A, Djian P, Potel JF, Hulet C, Jouve F, Bussière C, Ehkirch FP, Burdin G, Dubrana F, et al. Causes for failure of ACL reconstruction and influence of meniscectomies after revision. Knee Surg Sports Traumatol Arthrosc. 2011;19:196–201. https://doi.org/10.1007/s00167-010-1201-6.
182. Trojani C, Beaufi ls P, Burdin G, et al. Revision ACL reconstruction: infl uence of a lateral tenodesis. Knee Surg Sports Traumatol Arthrosc. 2012;20(8):1565–70.
183. Trojani C, Beaufils P, Burdin G, Bussière C, Chassaing V, Djian P, Dubrana F, Ehkirch FP, Franceschi JP, Hulet C, Jouve F. Revision ACL reconstruction: influence of a lateral tenodesis. Knee Surgery, Sports Traumatology, Arthroscopy. 2012 Aug;20:1565–70. https://doi.org/10.1007/s00167-011-1765-9
184. Tuphé P, Foissey C, Unal P, Vieira TD, Chambat P, Fayard JM, Thaunat M. Long-term natural history of unrepaired stable ramp lesions: a retrospective analysis of 28 patients with a minimum follow-up of 20 years. Am J Sports Med. 2022;50:3273–9. https://doi.org/10.1177/03635465221120058.
185. Uchio Y, Ochi M, Adachi N, Kawasaki K, Kuriwaka M. Determination of time of biologic fi xation after anterior cruciate ligament reconstruction with hamstring tendons. Am J Sports Med. 2003;31(3):345–52.
186. Vaishya R, Hasija R. Joint hypermobility and anterior cruciate ligament injury. J Orthopaed Surg. 2013;21:182–184. https://doi.org/10.1177/230949901302100213.
187. Vap AR, Persson A, Fenstad AM, Moatshe G, LaPrade RF, Engebretsen L. Re-revision anterior cruciate ligament reconstruction: an evaluation from the Norwegian knee ligament registry. Arthroscopy.

188. Vermeijden HD, Yang XA, van der List JP, DiFelice GS, Rademakers MV, Kerkhoffs GMMJ. Trauma and femoral tunnel position are the most common failure modes of anterior cruciate ligament reconstruction: a systematic review. Knee Surg Sports Traumatol Arthrosc. 2020;28:3666–75. https://doi.org/10.1007/s00167-020-06160-9.
189. Vertullo CJ, Quick M, Jones A, Grayson JE. A surgical technique using presoaked vancomycin hamstring grafts to decrease the risk of infection after anterior cruciate ligament reconstruction. Arthroscopy. 2012;28:337–42. https://doi.org/10.1016/j.arthro.2011.08.301.
190. Vrooijink SHA, Wolters F, Van Eck CF, Fu FH. Measurements of knee morphometrics using MRI and arthroscopy: a comparative study between ACL-injured and non-injured subjects. Knee Surg Sports Traumatol Arthrosc. 2011;19(Supplement 1):S12–6. https://doi.org/10.1007/s00167-011-1502-4.
191. Wang C, Lee YHD, Siebold R. Recommendations for the management of septic arthritis after ACL reconstruction. Knee Surg Sports Traumatol Arthrosc. 2014;22:2136–44. https://doi.org/10.1007/s00167-013-2648-z.
192. Webster KE, Feller JA, Leigh WB, Richmond AK. Younger patients are at increased risk for graft rupture and contralateral injury after anterior cruciate ligament reconstruction. Am J Sports Med. 2014 42 641–647. https://doi.org/10.1177/0363546513517540.
193. Weiler A, Schmeling A, Stohr I, Kaab MJ, Wagner M. Primary versus single-stage revision anterior cruciate ligament reconstruction using autologou hamstring tendon grafts: a prospective matched-group analysis. Am J Sports Med. 2007;35(10):1643–52.
194. Weiler A, Schmeling A, Stöhr I, Kääb MJ, Wagner M. Primary versus single- stage revision anterior cruciate ligament reconstruction using autologous hamstring tendon grafts: a prospective matched-group analysis. Am J Sports Med. 2007;35:1643–52. https://doi.org/10.1177/0363546507303114.
195. Werner BC, Gilmore CJ, Hamann JC, Gaskin CM, Carroll JJ, Hart JM, Miller MD. Revision anterior cruciate ligament reconstruction: results of a single-stage approach using allograft dowel bone grafting for femoral defects. J Am Acad Orthop Surg. 2016;24:581–7. https://doi.org/10.5435/JAAOS-D-15-00572.
196. Westermann RW, Wolf BR, Elkins J. Optimizing graft placement in anterior cruciate ligament reconstruction: a finite element analysis. J Knee Surg. 2017;30:97–106. https://doi.org/10.1055/s-0036-1581137.
197. Wiggins AJ, Grandhi RK, Schneider DK, Stanfield D, Webster KE, Myer GD. Risk of secondary injury in younger athletes after anterior cruciate ligament reconstruction: a systematic review and meta-analysis. Am J Sports Med. 2016;44:1861–76. https://doi.org/10.1177/0363546515621554.
198. Wilde J, Bedi A, Altchek DW. Revision anterior cruciate ligament reconstruction. Sports Health. 2014 Nov;6(6):504–18. https://doi.org/10.1177/1941738113500910. PMID: 25364483; PMCID: PMC4212350.
199. Wilson TC, Kantaras A, Atay A, Johnson DL. Tunnel enlargement after anterior cruciate ligament surgery. Am J Sports Med. 2004;32(2):543–9.
200. Wolf JM, Cameron KL, Owens BD. Impact of joint laxity and hypermobility on the musculoskeletal system. J Am Acad Orthop Surg. 2011;19:463–71. https://doi.org/10.5435/00124635-201108000-00002.
201. Won HH, Chang CB, Je MS, Chang MJ, Kim TK. Coronal limb alignment and indications for high tibial osteotomy in patients undergoing revision ACL reconstruction. Clin Orthopaed Relat Res. 2013;471:3504–3511. https://doi.org/10.1007/s11999-013-3185-2.
202. Woo SL, Hollis JM, Adams DJ, Lyon RM, Takai S. Tensile properties of the human femur-anterior cruciate ligament-tibia complex. The effects of specimen age and orientation. Am J Sports Med. 1991;19(3):217–225.
203. Wright RW, Huston LJ, Spindler KP, et al. Descriptive epidemiology of the Multicenter ACL Revision Study (MARS) cohort. Am J Sports Med. 2010;38(10):1979–86.
204. Wright RW, Preston E, Fleming BC, et al. A systematic review of anterior cruciate ligament reconstruction rehabilitation: part II: open versus closed kinetic chain exercises, neuromuscular electrical stimulation, accelerated rehabilitation, and miscellaneous topics. J Knee Surg. 2008;21(3):225–34.

205. Wright R, Spindler K, Huston L, et al. Revision ACL reconstruction outcomes: MOON cohort. J Knee Surg. 2011;24(4):289–94.
206. Xiao Y, Liang Z, Shen S, Liu F, Hu H, Chen B. Increased ACL direct insertion coverage provided more positive biomechanical effects on graft and bone tunnel during knee flexion: a simulation study. Journal of Experimental Orthopaedics 2023;10:108. https://doi.org/10.1186/s40634-023-00677-x
207. Yoon KH, Lee HW, Park JY, Kim SJ, Kim SG. Clinical outcomes and the failure rate of revision anterior cruciate ligament reconstruction were comparable between patients younger than 40 years and patients older than 40 years: a minimum 2-year follow-up study. Arthroscopy. 2020;36:2513–22. https://doi.org/10.1016/j.arthro.2020.06.012.
208. Yoshiya S, Kurosaka M, Ouchi K, Kuroda R, Mizuno K. Graft tension and knee stability after anterior cruciate ligament reconstruction. Clin Orthop Relat Res. 2002;394:154–60.
209. Zeng C, Cheng L, Wei J, Gao SG, Yang TB, Luo W, Li YS, Xu M, Lei GH. The influence of the tibial plateau slopes on injury of the anterior cruciate ligament: a meta- analysis. Knee Surg Sports Traumatol Arthrosc. 2014;22:53–65. https://doi.org/10.1007/s00167-012-2277-y.
210. Zhang ZY, Yin Y, Bai WB, Shi WL, Pan XY, Huang HJ, Zhang X, Wang C, Wang JQ. Association of Concomitant MRI-Determined Anterolateral Complex Injury With Quantitative Measurements of Altered Rotational Tibiofemoral Position on MRI in Patients With ACL Injury. Orthop J Sports Med. 2024 Feb 27;12(2):23259671241230954. https://doi.org/10.1177/23259671241230954. PMID: 38414665; PMCID: PMC10898314.
211. Zhao L, Lu M, Deng M, Xing J, He L, Wang C. Outcome of bone-patellar tendon- bone vs hamstring tendon autograft for anterior cruciate ligament reconstruction: a meta- analysis of randomized controlled trials with a 5-year minimum follow-up. Medicine 2020;99:e23476. https://doi.org/10.1097/MD.0000000000023476.
212. Zheng T, Song GY, Feng H, Zhang H, Li Y, Li X, Zhang ZJ, Ni QK, Feng Z. Lateral meniscus posterior root lesion influences anterior tibial subluxation of the lateral compartment in extension after anterior cruciate ligament injury. Am J Sports Med. 2020;48:838–46. https://doi.org/10.1177/0363546520902150.
213. Zhuo H, Pan L, Xu Y, Li J. Functional, magnetic resonance imaging, and Second- Look arthroscopic outcomes after pullout repair for avulsion tears of the posterior lateral meniscus root. Am J Sports Med. 2021;49:450–458. https://doi.org/10.1177/0363546520976635.

MIX
Papier aus verantwortungsvollen Quellen
Paper from responsible sources
FSC® C105338

If you have any concerns about our products,
you can contact us on
**ProductSafety@springernature.com**

In case Publisher is established outside the EU,
the EU authorized representative is:
**Springer Nature Customer Service Center GmbH**
**Europaplatz 3, 69115 Heidelberg, Germany**

Printed by Libri Plureos GmbH
in Hamburg, Germany